Periodontology - New Insights

Edited by Gokul Sridharan

Published in London, United Kingdom

Periodontology - New Insights
http://dx.doi.org/10.5772/intechopen.100796
Edited by Gokul Sridharan

Contributors
Rui Vitorino, Rita Ferreira, Sofia Guedes, Francisco Amado, Luís Perpétuo, Luiza Rusu, Renganath Murugan Jeyasree, Thamilselvan Muthuraj, Leela Subhashini C. Choudary Alluri, Pandu R. Gangula, David A. Mott, Chethan Sampath, Cherae Farmer-Dixon, Kristen Puckett, Kaitlyn Logan, Jazmyne Walker, Gerald Davis, Avishek Das, Debajyoti Mondal, Nam Cong-Nhat Huynh, Tracey Lynn Harney, Irina-Georgeta Sufaru, Maria-Alexandra Martu, Ionut Luchian, Silvia Teslaru, Simona Stoleriu, Stefan-Ioan Stratul, Darian Rusu, Monica Silvia Tatarciuc, Sorina Mihaela Solomon, Luis V. Maita-Véliz, Luis M. Maita-Castañeda, Nancy Srivastava, Shivendra Rana

First published in London, United Kingdom, 2023 by IntechOpen
IntechOpen is the global imprint of INTECHOPEN LIMITED, registered in England and Wales, registration number: 11086078, 5 Princes Gate Court, London, SW7 2QJ, United Kingdom
Printed in Croatia

British Library Cataloguing-in-Publication Data
A catalogue record for this book is available from the British Library

Additional hard and PDF copies can be obtained from orders@intechopen.com

Periodontology - New Insights
Edited by Gokul Sridharan
p. cm.

This title is part of the Dentistry Book Series, Volume 13
Topic: Oral Health
Series Editor: Sergio Alexandre Gehrke
Topic Editor: Sandra Marinho and Esra Guzeldemir-Akcakanat

Print ISBN 978-1-80356-992-5
Online ISBN 978-1-80356-993-2
eBook (PDF) ISBN 978-1-80356-994-9
ISSN 2631-6218

IntechOpen Book Series
Dentistry
Volume 13

Aims and Scope of the Series

This book series will offer a comprehensive overview of recent research trends as well as clinical applications within different specialties of dentistry. Topics will include overviews of the health of the oral cavity, from prevention and care to different treatments for the rehabilitation of problems that may affect the organs and/or tissues present. The different areas of dentistry will be explored, with the aim of disseminating knowledge and providing readers with new tools for the comprehensive treatment of their patients with greater safety and with current techniques. Ongoing issues, recent advances, and future diagnostic approaches and therapeutic strategies will also be discussed. This series of books will focus on various aspects of the properties and results obtained by the various treatments available, whether preventive or curative.

Meet the Series Editor

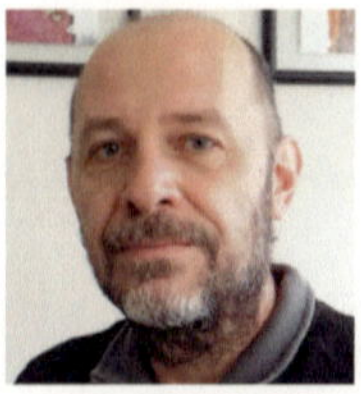

Dr. Sergio Alexandre Gehrke is a doctorate holder in two fields. The first is a Ph.D. in Cellular and Molecular Biology from the Pontificia Catholic University, Porto Alegre, Brazil, in 2010 and the other is an International Ph.D. in Bioengineering from the Universidad Miguel Hernandez, Elche/Alicante, Spain, obtained in 2020. In 2018, he completed a postdoctoral fellowship in Materials Engineering in the NUCLEMAT of the Pontificia Catholic University, Porto Alegre, Brazil. He is currently the Director of the Postgraduate Program in Implantology of the Bioface/UCAM/PgO (Montevideo, Uruguay), Director of the Cathedra of Biotechnology of the Catholic University of Murcia (Murcia, Spain), an Extraordinary Full Professor of the Catholic University of Murcia (Murcia, Spain) as well as the Director of the private center of research Biotecnos – Technology and Science (Montevideo, Uruguay). Applied biomaterials, cellular and molecular biology, and dental implants are among his research interests. He has published several original papers in renowned journals. In addition, he is also a Collaborating Professor in several Postgraduate programs at different universities all over the world.

Meet the Volume Editor

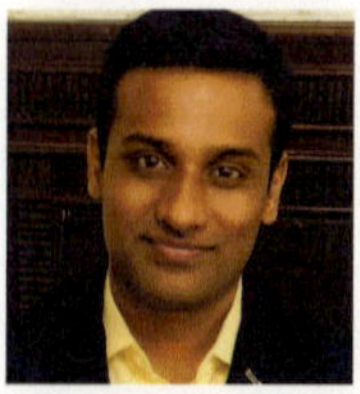

Dr. Gokul Sridharan is a professor in the Department of Oral Pathology and Microbiology at YMT Dental College and Hospital in Navi Mumbai. He completed his Ph.D. thesis on "Salivary and Serum Metabolomics in Oral Leukoplakia and Oral Squamous Cell Carcinoma." His research interests include oral pre-cancer, oral cancer, salivary diagnostics, oral and maxillofacial diseases, and advanced diagnostic aids, with a focus on bioinformatics and metabolomics. He has published several scientific papers and serves as a peer reviewer for numerous prestigious journals. Dr. Sridharan is also an active member of several journal editorial boards. He holds a diploma in medical law and ethics and is qualified in smoking cessation and control.

Contents

Preface

Oral diseases are a prevalent health issue, both communicable and non-communicable, that can cause pain, discomfort, disfigurement, and even death, posing a significant health burden for many countries. According to the WHO, almost 3.5 billion people worldwide are affected by oral diseases. This number may be even higher in developing countries, where a lack of awareness among the public, inadequate infrastructure, and limited access to oral healthcare providers, especially for individuals of lower socio-economic status, may contribute to increased prevalence. Periodontology is a specialized field of dentistry that deals with the health and disease of the periodontium, which includes the teeth and their supporting structures. The maintenance of a healthy periodontium is crucial for preserving dentition integrity. Over the years, there have been several essential advances in the pathophysiology, classification, diagnosis, and management of periodontal disease.

This book aims to provide researchers and clinicians with an overview of the most recent insights regarding the periodontium and periodontal diseases. The book contains various chapters that cover newer diagnosis and treatment modalities, as well as contributing to the understanding of the molecular aspects of periodontal disease.

Gokul Sridharan, MDS, Ph.D., PGD (Medical Law and Ethics)
Department of Oral Pathology and Microbiology,
Dr. G. D. Pol Foundation YMT Dental College and Hospital,
Navi Mumbai, India

Chapter 1

The Salivary Secretome

Luís Perpétuo, Rita Ferreira, Sofia Guedes, Francisco Amado and Rui Vitorino

Abstract

Recently, proteomics has emerged as an important tool for understanding biological systems, protein–protein interactions, and networks that ultimately lead to a deeper understanding of the underlying mechanisms of certain diseases. More recently, the study of secretomes, a type of proteomics, has also been highlighted as a potential next step in the field of diagnosis/prognosis. The secretome is the set of proteins expressed by an organism and secreted into the extracellular space, comprising 13–20% of all proteins. Since almost all, if not all, organs produce secretomes, this means that it is possible to study secretomes and trace these proteins back to their origin, supporting the idea that this could indeed be very important in diagnosing certain diseases. This is often combined with techniques such as mass spectrometry to measure the secretome of, for example, a particular tissue, and bioinformatics tools and databases to give us an idea of what to expect (prediction). In this paper, we will give a general overview of this world, but with a focus on the new bioinformatics tools and databases, their advantages and disadvantages, as well as a deeper look at isolation systems for proteomes, specifically salivary secretomes. Indeed, the salivary secretome represents a valuable new tool capable of providing insights into immunopathology and potentially aiding in diagnostics. Furthermore, we will explore applications of these methods and give an idea of what the future holds for such promising techniques: Salivary secretome in conjunction with bioinformatics tools/databases in the diagnosis of diseases (such as diabetes, Sjogren's syndrome, and cardiovascular disease).

Keywords: Saliva, bioinformatic tools, prediction

1. Introduction

Salivary plasma is also known as ultrafiltrate of biological fluid. Nearly 1,000 different proteins and 19,000 unique peptide sequences have been found in saliva. Whole saliva (WMS) is a combination of various secretions produced by major and minor salivary glands, gingiva cervical fluid (GCF), mucosal transmission, oral wound serum and blood vessels [1].

Saliva is mainly composed of three main pairs of salivary glands, namely the parotid gland, the sublingual gland, and the lingual gland. Saliva is composed of 99.5% water, 0.3% protein and 0.2% trace elements. The concentration of proteins and peptides in saliva is very important for the maintenance of oral health and homeostasis. The increased frequency and severity of oral diseases are often related to changes in salivary protein content [2, 3]. Salivary proteins facilitate food perception and digestion, maintain the integrity of mineralized tooth and oral epithelial surfaces, shield the oral digestive tract from environmental hazards and invading pathogens, and protect oral tissues from fungal or viral infections [4, 5]. Moreover, it is suggested that the origins of salivary proteins can be analyzed throughout mixed saliva and that post-transcriptional modifications may play a key role in understanding secretome network pathways [6, 7]. Moreover, Feizi et al., 2020 [7] found that the study of secretion pathways (translocation, folding, trafficking and glycosylation) is relevant to know tissue-specific secretion pathways and tissue-specific secretomes that would facilitate the elaboration of a link between proteins and diseases.

Salivary gland secretome represents a valuable new tool to measure many local soluble mediators to gain future insight into immunopathology and potentially aid in diagnosis [8]. This method could be of use to identify therapeutic targets and develop markers for stratification, prognosis and treatment response in patients [9, 10].

Biomarkers are defined as biological molecules found in blood, saliva, and other body fluids, as symptoms of normal or abnormal processes, or symptoms of conditions or diseases. Few studies have demonstrated the relationship between serum and saliva levels of clinically used biomarkers. Nevertheless, human saliva has attracted attention as a liquid biopsy for the diagnosis of oral diseases as a potential target. Salivary biomarkers are used for evaluation, prediction and diagnosis of various diseases. They can be collected rapidly in a non-invasive, natural and painless way. Salivary research can help identify biomarkers associated with health and disease conditions [1, 11, 12]. Collection and storage of saliva is also simple, relatively cheap and low risk for patients and healthcare professionals [3, 13, 14]. Salivary proteomics is a promising tool as proteomic molecules control the direct antibacterial action of microorganisms in the oral cavity, but has limitations including non-applicability in the driest patients and technical challenges such as the degradation of cytokines by salivary enzymes [9]. Optimization of existing histology protocols to determine salivary gland inflammation will help improve the diagnosis of various diseases [9, 10].

2. Definition

Under both normal and pathological conditions, cells secrete a variety of proteins into the extracellular space via classical and non-classical secretory pathways [5]. The majority of these proteins represent the pathophysiology of the cell from which they are secreted. Recently, although more than 92% of protein-coding genes have been mapped by the Human Proteome Map Project, a large number of these proteins that constitute the cell's secretome is still unknown [4].

Secreted proteins or the secretome may be accessible in body fluids and are therefore considered as potential biomarkers to distinguish between healthy and diseased individuals [8]. To facilitate biomarker discovery and further assist clinicians and scientists working in these areas, we compiled and cataloged secreted proteins from the human proteome using an integrated bioinformatics approach [9, 10]. In this study, it was found that nearly 14% of the human proteome is likely secreted via classical and non-classical secretion pathways. Of these, ~38% of these secreted proteins were found in extracellular vesicles including exosomes and shedding microvesicles.

Of these secreted proteins, 94% were detected in human body fluids including blood, plasma, serum, saliva, semen, tears, and urine. We hypothesize that this list of secreted proteins with high confidence could serve as a compendium of biomarker candidates. In addition, the catalog could provide functional insights into understanding the molecular mechanisms involved in various physiological and pathophysiological conditions.

The highly elevated inflammatory mediators in the secretions of patients with complex diseases such as primary Sjögren's syndrome (PSS) are related to clinical parameters.

2.1 Secreted proteins

A secreted protein can be defined as a protein that is actively transported outside the cell. In humans, cells such as endocrine cells and B lymphocytes are specialized in the secretion of proteins, most cells secrete proteins in different. Not only is this a rich source of new treatments and drug targets, but most of the blood diagnostic tests used in the clinic target secreted proteins, underscoring the importance of these proteins to medicine and biology. These include pancreatic enzymes (PRSS1, CELA3A, AMY2A) and other digestive enzymes expressed in the salivary glands (PRR4, STATH, ZG16B) or stomach (PGA3, PGA4). The liver is one of the most important secretory organs and produces high amounts of plasma proteins such as albumin, fibrinogen and transferrin. Another group of highly secreted proteins belongs to the diphenhydramine family and is secreted by glandular cells in the epididymis (DEFB118, DEFB106A and DEFB129).

2.2 Membrane proteins

Membrane proteins are one of the largest and most important classes of proteins. Membrane proteins are associated with cell membranes or organs in cells and can be classified as peripheral or integrated. Peripheral membrane proteins bind to the membrane by binding to the peripheral region of the membrane or by integrated membrane proteins, but cannot completely penetrate the membrane. Integrated membrane proteins have a hydrophobic α-helical or β-barrel structure so that they can be distributed throughout the lipid molecule and linked by the outer loop region of the membrane. The α-helical integral membrane protein is the main type of membrane protein and is found in all types of biological membranes. This explains why their key roles as transporters and receptors currently account for about 57% of approved drug targets, as they are of great importance to the pharmaceutical industry. Many important receptors and cell surface molecules are found in the list of human cell differentiation molecules (CD markers). The G protein synthesis receptor (GPCR) comprises seven transmembrane fragments (DM) and contains 775 human protein-coding genes, making it the largest membrane protein target.

2.3 Classification of the human proteome

Despite the availability of the human salivary proteome, the origin of individual proteins remains unclear. So far, more than 3000 proteins have been identified in various studies, and with new tools and methods, more will be identified [4].

Meinken et al., 2015 [15] analyzed the subcellular location of the protein using MetazSecKB. The subcellular location of the protein is an important factor that determines the function of the protein molecule in the organism. MetazSecKB is a knowledge base for subcellular proteins developed specifically for metazoans (i.e., humans and animals). More than 4 million protein sequence data entries have been retrieved from UniProt, including 121 complete proteins. The location of protein subgroups, including secretion and 15 subgroup sites, are assigned based on selected test evidence or predictions using 7 computational tools [15].

Various identifiers, gene names, keywords and types can be used to search and download protein or subcellular protein data. Support BLAST search and community annotation of sublocalizations. Our preliminary analysis shows that protein levels, secretome levels, and other subcellular protein levels vary widely among different animal species. Confidentiality levels range from 3–22% (mean 8%) in Metazzoa species [15].

Approximately 21–43% (mean 31%) in cytoplasm, 20–37% (mean 30%) in embryo, 3–19% (mean 12%) plasma membrane proteins and 3–9% (mean 6%) in mitochondria. The authors also compared protein families in different animal species [15]. Genetic oncology of human secreted proteins and field analysis of protein families show that these proteins play an important role in the development of human structure, signal transduction and regulation of many biological processes in the immune system [15].

The combination of the results of membrane protein and secretion analysis draws the distribution map of potential membrane proteins and secreted proteins in human membrane proteins. Three types are used to annotate the protein isoforms of all human genes: (i) secreted type, (ii) membrane type, and (iii) endogenous type (i.e., proteins with no predictable SP/TM properties). Note that proteins classified as membranous may be localized in the endoplasmic reticulum or in the inner membrane, such as the colon. Each human protein-coding gene is classified as having all isoforms encoding protein isoforms belonging to one or two or three types of these groups. The results showed that at least 36% of the predicted human genes contain membrane-disseminated or secreted protein isoforms.

2.4 The plasma proteome

Plasma is the transparent, liquid part of blood that is formed when white blood cells, red blood cells, and platelets are removed. It consists of small substances such as water (90%), protein (7–8%), salt, gas, and nutrients. Plasma proteins contain up to 90% of the ten most abundant proteins, including albumin, fibrinogen, which is involved in blood clotting, and immunoglobulin, which is mainly involved in immune processes. One of the most important functions of plasma is to transport essential compounds to different parts of the body, regulate osmotic pressure and fluid exchange in all tissues, and play an important role in immune system function. Most cells in the body interact with plasma directly or indirectly through other fluids. Therefore, analysis of plasma proteins can provide important information about the patient's health status.

The dynamic range of plasma protein between the high albumin (ALB) concentration is more than 10 orders of magnitude. It has an extraordinary dynamic range. It can serve as a transporter and helps maintain the osmotic pressure of emulsification. Rare proteins containing interleukins are found in tissues. Although many proteins in the plasma proteome pass through the secretory pathway, there is another type of tissue-secreted proteins that are found in cells but can be released into plasma due to cell death or damage. There is also an interesting class of proteins that do not enter the ER/Golgi pathway by non-classical secretion and include cytokines such as interleukin 10 (IL10) and mitogens such as fibroblast growth factor 2 (FGF2).

2.5 The secretory pathway

In the secretory pathway, the signal sequence protein travels from the endoplasmic reticulum (ER) through the vesicles of the ER to the cell surface. The signal sequence that drives protein secretion is called a signal peptide. It is a short hydrophobic N-terminus that is inserted into the ER membrane and separated from the protein. In most cases, the N-terminal transmembrane (TM) acts as part of the signal line. The ER signal sequence is recognized by the chaperone protein, which guides the ribosome to the approximate ER where transfer of the protein sequence takes place in a protein complex called the translocon. The membrane protein is transferred by the translocation protein to the lipid player of the ER membrane, and the secreted protein is transferred into the lumen of ER. Proteins that pass the quality control of ER are transported by vesicles to the Golgi, where they are further modified in important processes such as glycosylation and phosphorylation. The Golgi is also responsible for sorting proteins for transport to their final destination. These proteins are usually plasma membranes, lysosomes or cell secretions.

3. Systems for isolation

With the use of novel advanced technologies, many oral and systemic diseases can be treated early with non-invasive, easy to follow, time-saving and personalized solutions, further enhancing the potential of salivary secretome [16].

3.1 Common methods used to identify salivary secretome

Salivary secretome mainly includes proteins, metabolites, genes, microorganisms and immune system. Various methods are used to analyze molecules to study and verify biomarkers. Proteins can be used to diagnose diabetes, periodontitis, dental caries and AIDS [16, 17]. However, salivary transcriptome and genes include mRNA and DNA. Genetic chip sequencing, DNA hybridization, qPCR and gel electrophoresis help in identifying various diseases. On the other hand, metabolic research requires and uses gas chromatography–mass spectrometry, nuclear magnetic resonance spectroscopy and high-performance liquid chromatography. These methods can be used to diagnose diabetes, lung cancer, pancreatic cancer, breast cancer and Sjogren's syndrome [17, 18].

3.2 Saliva biomarker-based platforms

The analysis system is based on different technologies used to detect biomarkers in saliva. Single and multiple systems (e.g. MEMS, ORI, chromatographic test strips and multiple salivary glands (US)) are only used to detect proteins and whole proteins and nucleic acids (e.g. IL -8, MMP-8, α-amylase, e.g. IV, HCV) up to 1 minute [19], and there is a short time limit. Therefore, these technologies have reduced the aggressive behavior to a higher level [19].

3.3 Novel isolation techniques

Biosensor is a biological analyzer that can replicate any biological material. The biosensor works by biometrically identifying specific components and is designed for target analysis. They remain selective and sensitive to the presence of other interfering compounds. In the medical field, the application of biosensors is growing rapidly [20, 21]. They can detect antibodies/antigens, nucleic acids, cell structures or enzymes. The transducers can be electrochemical, thermometric, optical, piezoelectric or magnetic.

3.4 Automated mass spectrometry-based approach

Using liquid chromatography–tandem mass spectrometry (LC -MS/MS) to identify novel targets in specially prepared cell secretions, Wetie et al., 2013 [22] have developed an automated, simple and effective strategy. In addition, the supporting role of mass spectrometry (MS) in the functional evaluation of the identified secreted targets is investigated [22].

Simplicity is achieved by culturing cells in serum-free medium, which eliminates the need to remove large amounts of serum protein while minimizing unsightly matrix effects. Once these factors have been determined, their verification and nature is followed. In addition, this method can lead to the identification of abnormally secreted, spilled or exaggerated proteins in response to stimuli [22].

3.5 BioMEMS

The lab-on-a-chip system uses small and easy-to-build BioMEMS devices to detect biological and chemical agents. They are based on micro/nano scale fabrication systems and help to improve the sensitivity of sensor results. It has unlabeled detection technology including microconverter, surface plasmon oscillation and organic field effect transistors [23, 24].

Biological Micro-Electro-Mechanical Systems (MEMS) can be used in many applications, such as drug delivery, heart MEMS, hearing aids, insulin microbumps, endoscopic lens agents, and retinal prostheses for monitoring patients with heart disease [25].

3.6 Fluorescent biosensors

Fluorescent biosensors can be used in cancer, drug development, arthritis, cardiovascular and viral infections, chronic myeloid leukemia, etc. Efficient screening methods, applications of fluorescence studies in gene expression, protein location in cell cycle, cell apoptosis, signal transduction and transcription [26]. Nanomaterials and nanoproducts for biosensors offer opportunities for the next generation of biosensing. They can be widely used for monitoring, diagnosis, control and analysis [27].

3.7 Electrical field-induced release and measurement (EFIRM)

The liquid biopsy technique called EFIRM uses electrochemical methods to promote hybridization of nucleic acids [28]. This method enables precise detection of RNA and protein biomarker targets on exosomes. EFIRM can analyze mutation status within one hour without extracting DNA. It can detect cancer in oral cavity cancer, non-squamous lung cancer and epidermal growth factor (EGFR) mutations [29].

3.8 Microfluidics

Microfluidic applications work with integrated micromachining and specific physical and chemical properties. Originally, silicone, mineral glass and ceramics were used. These materials were replaced by soft and hard thermostatic and thermoplastic materials or biodegradable hydrogel materials.

The paper analytical device (μPADs) was first developed by Whiteside. Paper is microscopic and hydrophilic, so it provides the basis for the formation of microscopic channels. They are used to diagnose urine metabolism, blood glucose, pH, liver function and infectious agents [30].

4. Interaction with other systems

Saliva is a potential diagnostic tool that can provide a simple diagnostic method. The presence of salivary biomarkers can aid in early diagnosis. Saliva has the potential to revolutionize next-generation molecular testing. It can diagnose oral cancer, dental inflammation and periodontitis [31]. To date, many salivary biomarkers have been proposed for the diagnosis of oral cancer. Conventional medical standards are not sufficient to easily determine the location of active disease or to easily measure the progress of future disease. Genetic testing offers the most effective way to prevent dental disease in the long term [31–33].

In addition, several research groups have reported the use of whole saliva or glandular saliva for mass spectrometry-based proteomics research. The extensive enumeration of salivary proteins is done by combining the previous LC -MS/MS -based saliva research data with our research data [34].

Using the bioinformatics tools mentioned above, a possible analysis of gene ontology classification and their secretion was performed. Comparing with the latest human salivary proteins synthesized from oral cancer tissues expressing different proteins, we found proteins associated with oral cancer. The protein peptides of these proteinsor the most observed peptides were selected from the Global Protein Machine Database (GPMDP) [35].

5. Bioinformatics tools for secretome prediction

Proteins can flow from blood to salivary glands by active transport, passive diffusion, or ultrafiltration, and then some of them are released into saliva, so if accurately identified, they can be used as biomarkers of disease [36]. Researchers have developed a series of novel computational and biological communication tools to predict salivary biomarkers [37].

The basis of the prediction is a set of physicochemical and hierarchical features found between human proteins that can pass from blood to saliva and proteins that are not present in saliva [36, 37]. In 2013, Wang et al., [38] predicted human salivary proteins from blood and evaluated their use in identifying diagnostic biomarkers. This predictive capability can be used to predict potential biomarker proteins for specific human diseases, information about various exposed proteins in diseased and healthy control tissues, and the prognostic potential of proteins secreted in blood. This enables the use of antibody-based technology to target effective biomarkers in saliva. They used this comprehensive data to predict that 31 candidate biomarker proteins in saliva could be used in breast cancer [38].

5.1 Bioinformatic tools

Continued method development supports the comprehensive identification and quantification of secreted proteins at specific cellular levels. The role of secretory factors in regulating important signaling events has been discussed, and a connectivity diagram has been constructed to describe differential secretory expression and dynamic changes [39].

Bioinformatics has become a bridge between confidential data and computer tasks to manage, mine and retrieve information. Based on this information, predictions can be made to help clarify the physiological state of a particular organism and determine the specific dysfunction at the stage of disease. The major challenge in data analysis lies within the integration of biological information from different sources. Database enhancements and software improvements can greatly increase the practicality and reliability of confidential investigations [39]. Reliable data interpretation is essential for the formation and exploration of relevant disease biomarker proposals as well as the discovery of new drug targets. Using genetic oncology (GO), it is possible to collect basic information about secretome proteins. GO analysis can determine how the identified components relate to specific functions or processes and whether a particular type of protein is found in secretions. In addition, in a statistical framework, the method GO can determine whether there is an obvious GO period [40]. In the database GO, molecular functions are defined as the biochemical functions of gene products. The biological pathway refers to the integration of the biochemical properties of proteins. Pathway analysis is an important step to properly understand the uniqueness and function of secrets. Methods have been developed to assess whether protein packaging is present in the target phenotype. Using different tools, according to different group rules, can provide different and sometimes complementary information. The results are strongly influenced by the criteria chosen to define the target protein and the reference list [40, 41].

Ingenuity Path Analysis (IPA) and Meta Core (Genico) are commercial software for visualizing high performance data in a biological network environment. STRING is a free database of known and predicted protein interactions, including direct (physical) and indirect (functional) associations from various sources [42]. In this way, the network of protein–protein interaction, metabolism or genetic regulation can be reconstructed based on prior knowledge and the biological network can be reconstructed. Determined by the interaction between its components [42, 43].

Pathway analysis tools become very popular and can interpret omics data quickly. To date, IPA has been highly cited in the field of proteomics, having been used in 121 publications. The software is designed to interpret large genetic datasets, but it can also be used to illustrate the biological implications of complex proteomics datasets [43].

Data sharing presents a new challenge for modern proteomics. The first obstacle to data sharing is the data format. Each MS tool generates a file from the source data in a proprietary format. The HUPO-PSI standard has been accepted by vendors and public web-based resource providers. The proteomics community has developed guidelines to facilitate storage and open access to proteomics data in a central public repository [44–46].

PeptideAtlas, PRIDE and Trench have been developed to share data among the entire proteomics research community [47–49]. Recently, the Proteome Change Alliance has established a place where MS proteomics data can be submitted to the existing major proteomics databases. The purpose is to facilitate data transfer between them to achieve the best data transfer and to create a global accession number for all participating databases. This information will be available to all MS/MS researchers in the UK who wish to use it for their research [47–49].

Using the innovative majority voting methods, Rehman et al., 2020, analyzed transcriptome data from 5 cancer types and more than 3000 samples to measure the relative difference in gene expression of secretory proteins compared to normal tissue in the vicinity. A comprehensive, in-depth data mining analysis reveals that among several cancer types, a continuous group of uncontrolled secretory protein subtypes is concentrated in hematopoietic cell lines. Genes associated with hematopoietic cell lineages are often reduced during the continuous development of cancer, and high exposure levels are associated with good prognosis for patients [50].

Moreover, they suggest that cancer cells suppress the underlying mechanism of hematopoietic cell lineage signaling by reducing the expression of immune-related genes. The data identify potential biomarkers for cancer immunotherapy. It can be concluded that this method is applicable to define other cancers and highlight specific targets for treatment and diagnosis [50].

5.2 BONCAT and pulsed SILAC

Despite the increasing interest in secretomes associated with paracrine/autocrine mechanisms, mass spectrometric cell studies have been performed using serum-free media (SFM). On the other hand, the use of serum culture medium (SCM) is not necessarily recommended because secretions obtained with SCM are easily contaminated with fetal serum proteins (FBS) [51].

Shin et al., 2019, [51] used biological non-designated amino acid tags (BONCAT) and pulsed SILAC (pSILAC) to analyze the different secreted proteins between SFM and SCM. Mesenchymal stem cells are derived from human cancer cells U87MG and human Wharton's Jelly (hWJ-MSCs) [51]. In most cases, the biological communication equipment predicts that the protein is secreted when the protein secretion level in SCM is higher than in SFM. In HWJ-MSC, the amount of protein secreted in SCM within 24 hours, even considering different cell proliferation rates, is greater than SFM [51]. The highly secreted HWJ-MSC protein in SCM contains many positive markers of angiogenesis, neurogenesis and osteogenesis, as well as MSc-paracrine factors involved in upstream regulators of cell proliferation. This result indicates that secretome analysis should be processed in SCM to promote cell proliferation and secretion [51].

Another computational method was evaluated by Min, 2010 [52] to understand the prediction accuracy of signal B, phobia, target B and wolf sport, which can be used alone or in combination with DMHMM and PS scanning. Prediction accuracy is represented by Mathews Correlation Coefficient (MCC). Tools for predicting proteins secreted in different eukaryotic kingdoms show different advantages. Using his own tools, the author found Wolfsport for fungi (73.1%), Phobius for animals (82.8%), Signal B for plants (55.4%) and Phobius for proteases (42.1%) [52].

The use of TMHMM significantly improves the prediction accuracy of all datasets. According to the measured accuracy, it is recommended to use the following methods to make secret predictions for different eukaryotes: signal P/DMHM/wolfport/Phobius/PS scan for fungi (83.4%), Phobius/wolfb/animal/PS -86A Phobius/target P/PS scan (73.2%), combined with all tools for protists (52.8%) [52].

Free interactive resources are provided within the portal Human Protein Atlas (www.proteinatlas.org) and analyzed by Uhlén et al., 2015 [53]. The portal offers the possibility to explore tissue-expressed proteins in tissues and organs and to analyze tissue profiles for specific protein classes. A large list of proteins expressed at high levels in different tissues was compiled to localize the protein in the subunits of each tissue and organ and provide a spatial environment down to the level of individual cells [53].

6. Applications

Saliva is a complex fluid containing various enzymes, electrolytes, proteins, nucleic acids, antibacterial components, hormones, cytokines, and antibodies.

Its composition almost reflects the overall state of physical health and disease. It can become a diagnostic tool for many diseases. The submandibular saliva of patients with cystic fibrosis contains 66% more lipids per 100 milliliters of saliva than healthy substances. Salivary fatty acid profile can be used as a good indicator for early detection of heart disease. Dietary fat intake influences the increased arachidonic acid production associated with lung inflammation and heart disease.

Under normal and pathological conditions, cells secrete various types of proteins into the extracellular space via classical and nonclassical secretory pathways. Most of these proteins represent cell secretion pathologies. Recently, Human Protein Atlas Project has localized more than 92% of protein-coding genes, but the number of proteins secreted by cells is still difficult to determine [54]. Secreted proteins or secretions can enter body fluids and are therefore considered as potential biomarkers to distinguish healthy and diseased individuals. To facilitate the discovery of biomarkers and to further assist physicians and scientists working in this field, Keerthikumar et al., 2016, [54] used integrated bioinformatics methods to compile and list the secreted proteins in humans.

In this study, it was found that about 14% of human proteins can be secreted through classical and non-classical secretion pathways. Among them, about 38% of secreted proteins are in extracellular cells, including exosomes and excretory microorganisms. Of these secreted proteins, 94% are present in human body fluids, including blood, plasma, serum, saliva, semen, tears, and urine [54]. The author hypothesizes that this list of secreted proteins can serve as a set of candidate biomarkers with high confidence. They can provide functional insights to understand the molecular mechanisms associated with various physiological and pathophysiological states of cells [54].

Chen et al., 2019, [55] found that secretory proteins are widely expressed in various tissues and body fluids, and a large proportion of them are expressed in a tissue-specific manner. In addition, there are 14 cancer-related secretory proteins. Their expression levels are significantly correlated with survival rates of patients with eight different tumors, which may be potential prognostic biomarkers [55]. Surprisingly, of the 6,943 secretory proteins, 89.21% (2,927 novel secretory proteins) have known protein domains [55]. The authors enriched these novel secretory proteins mainly by known domains related to immunity (such as immunoglobulin V set and C1 set domains). Their comprehensive novel secretory proteins and features provide insight into human confidentiality and are valuable resources for future research [55].

In Sjogren's syndrome, salivary flow is impaired due to tubular changes caused by lymphocyte infiltration and salivary gland fibrosis, and the patient suffers from toothache, infectious dysphagia, and other oral complaints. The blood lipid level of Sjogren's patients is twice that of normal healthy people, and the antibody level is high. Patients with Sjogren's syndrome or radiation therapy for head and neck cancer have severe dry mouth, which greatly affects their oral health and quality of life. Since there is no clinically proven treatment, clinical management of xerostomia is limited to preventive treatment. Previous research has shown that mesenchymal stem cells (MMSC) derived from mouse bone marrow differ from salivary progenitors when grown together with mouse salivary epithelial cells [56]. Restrictive transcription factors in co-grown MMSCs are identified with amylase (AMY1), muscarinic 3 receptors (M3R), aquaporin 5 (AQP5), tubular morphological changes, and acinar cell marker expression [56]. This cell marker is called cytokeratin 19 (CK19). Mona et al., 2020, investigated inducible molecules in a conditioned medium that can trigger MMSC replication and integrated mass spectrometry and systems biology by high

Bioinformatic tool/database	Features	Accessibility	Website
BIOCARTA	Protein-pathway association	B	https://maayanlab-cloud/Harmonizome/dataset/Biocarta+Pathways
BLAST	Sequence similarities comparison	C	https://blast.ncbi.nlm.nih.gov/Blast.cgi
DisGeNET	Gene and variability associated with disease	B	https://www.disgenet.org/
Gene Ontology	Computational model of biological systems (genes)	A	http://geneontology.org/
GPM	Proteomics data analysis, reuse and validation for biological and biomedical research	C	https://www.thegpm.org/
IPA	Genomic and clinical knowledge	A	https://digitalinsights.qiagen.com/
KEGG	Database of high-level functions on biological systems	C	https://www.genome.jp/kegg/
Meta Core	Omics analysis	B	https://portal.genego.com/
MetazSecKBGene	Knowledgebase for human/animal secretomes	B	http://proteomics.ysu.edu/secretomes/animal/index.php
Panther	Biological pathways	B	http://www.pantherdb.org/
PathwayStudio	Network between omics and biological processes	A	https://www.pathwaystudio.com/
PeptideAtlas	MS/MS peptide data	B	http://www.peptideatlas.org/
Philius	Signal peptide prediction	A	http://wwwyeastrc.org/philius/pages/philius/runPhilius.jsp
Phobius	Signal peptide prediction	B	http://phobius.sbc-su.se/
PRIDE	Proteomics datasets	B	http://www.ebi-ac.uk/pride/
SecretomeP	Non-classical secretion prediction	A	http://www.cbs.dtu.dk/services/SecretomeP/
SignalP	Signal peptide prediction	A	http://www.cbs.dtu.dk/services/SignalP/
STRING	Protein–protein interaction networks	A	https://string-db.org/
TMHMM	Transmembrane helix prediction	A	http://www.cbs.dtu.dk/services/TMHMM/
UniProt	Protein database	B	http://www.uniprot.org/
Wolfpsort	Subcellular localization prediction	B	https://wolfpsort.hgc.ip/

A - easy to use and accessible, B - accessible but hard to use, C - hard to access and use.

Table 1.
Bioinformatics tools and databases that predict secreted proteins.

performance liquid chromatography. Based on their key roles in embryonic development and salivary gland growth, our method identified ten differentially expressed proteins [56]. In addition, systems biology analysis revealed six candidate proteins, namely cysteine-rich insulin-like growth factor binding protein 7 (IgFPP7), pro-angiogenic stimulant 61 (CYR61), acrin (AGRN), laminin, beta 2 (LAMP2), folistatin 1 (FSDL1) and fibronectin 1 (FN1), all of which could potentially contribute to the propagation of MMSC during co-cultivation [56].

Human salivary secretome plays a diagnostic role in the diagnosis of heart disease. Diabetes is another common disease that is rapidly developing worldwide. Due to its non-invasiveness, cheap and simple saliva samples are attractive as diagnostic fluids for diabetes analysis. The announced study concluded that various biomarkers are used in the early stages to diagnose diabetes. Compared to serum of diabetic and diabetic patients, salivary glucose, amylase, calcium, phosphorus and calcium levels show significant changes.

Salivary secretome test requires proper identification and verification of biomarkers. Diagnosis and biomarkers are measurable parameters that can interact physiologically and biochemically at the molecular or cellular level and always serve as normal indicators. The pathology and intervention behavior of the human body can be identified using biomarkers present in salivary secretome. Biomarkers include many categories, such as protein, DNA, RNA, metabolism and microorganisms, so they are all used together (**Table 1**).

7. Future perspectives

With our current results, we note that although the secretome has gained attention and has been highlighted in recent studies, it is still of interest to explore this topic more deeply. In future studies, we propose to go beyond the usual protein profiling and perform network studies to find links between proteins from salivary secretome in direct and indirect ways. In addition, studies have begun to evaluate the role that transcriptional and post-transcriptional modifications of proteins have in informing their origin [6, 7]. This will be relevant for establishing links between salivary protein levels and disease prognosis/diagnosis.

In **Figure 1**, we see a flowchart of the information presented in this paper. Starting from a secretome: how do we detect it (detection approach), how do we identify it (protein identification), how do we verify information about these proteins (record repositories and inventory of the secretome). This line of work leads to the analysis of the secretome, but makes up only part of the pipeline. Prediction tools are also of great use (genomic datasets enable the existence of tools to predict secretory proteins). Several of the bioinformatics tools discussed previously can be used to perform secretome analysis, where we can limit the investigation to protein profiling, but also go beyond that to investigate signaling pathways, networks (protein–protein, gene-protein, protein-disease), and determine useful disease biomarkers. All of this information culminates in getting closer to the biological significance of certain proteins and interactions under certain circumstances. **Figure 1** shows several examples of biomarkers mentioned in this review and narrows that down to applications for saliva testing, namely in areas such as prognosis and diagnosis. In summary, **Figure 1** represents the pipeline and workflow of secretome studies.

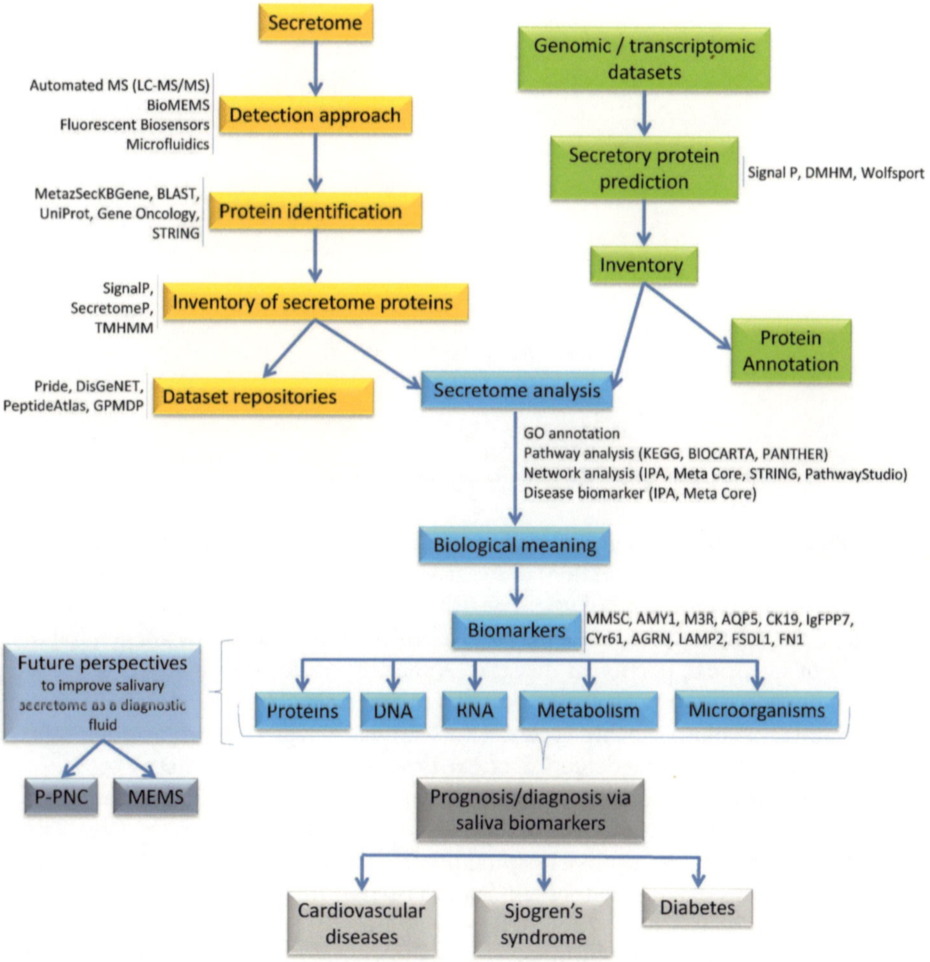

Figure 1.
Workflow of secretome analysis for the comprehensive characterization of molecules secreted by salivary glands, arriving at the final point (biomarkers) that can be used for prognosis/diagnosis in several diseases.

8. Conclusion

Although there are some limitations, salivary proteomics is a promising diagnostic and therapeutic tool for several critical diseases. Salivary gland secretome represents a valuable new tool to measure many local soluble mediators, provide future insight into immunopathology, and potentially aid in diagnosis.

Routine laboratory tests include hematology, clinical chemistry, and immunochemistry using high performance equipment. Diagnosis based on salivary secretome may provide an efficient, rapid and simple automated method for transformation. The next decade will bring improvements in accuracy, performance, and bed monitoring, but not hospital systems.

Improving basic healthcare systems with personalized medications, biosensors, lab-on-a-chip systems, personal genetics, and smartphone tracking parameters. The impact of saliva testing on healthcare systems is enormous, aggressive and convenient.

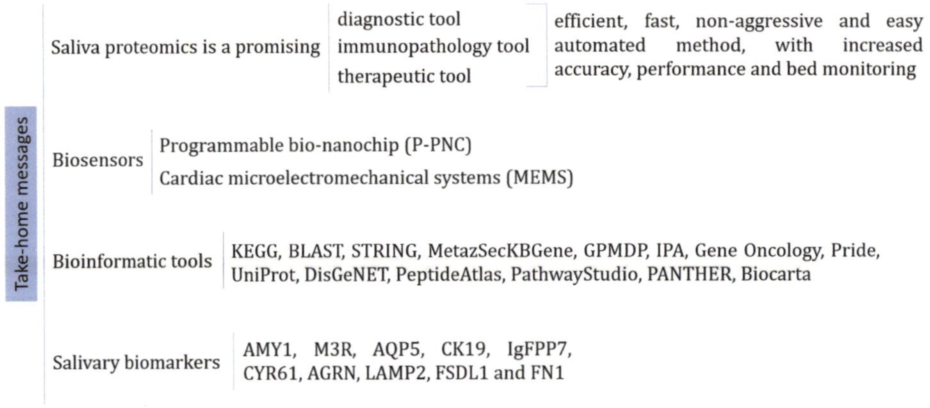

Figure 2.
Take-home messages that summarize the main ideas/concepts of this paper.

Reportedly, the ability to use saliva for a liquid biopsy is an important diagnostic tool for medical conditions and dental diseases. The simple model has information related to non-aggression and physical health, making it an attractive choice.

Some of the salivary secretome markers mentioned in this review are general markers, not specific to particular diseases. A more specific set of markers is needed to make salivary secretome an acceptable diagnostic fluid. The recent introduction of the programmable bio-nanochip system (P-PNC) has driven the revolution in saliva detection technology for the detection of cardiovascular disease (CVD).

Other biosensing systems, such as cardiac microelectromechanical systems (MEMS), can also be used to detect certain diseases. With the help of the latest labs in chip systems, they will improve hospital practice and human health [57]. Future development of this diagnostic tool will lead to further improvements in certain devices that will change the method of screening for critical diseases such as CVD.

A take-home message that summarizes, as shown in **Figure 2**, the main issues that have been addressed so far in salivary proteomics as a diagnostic and therapeutic tool. It also includes the means of detection and prediction of salivary proteomics (biosensors and bioinformatics tools). Although some have been used for a long time, most are novel tools and techniques that have been shown to provide great data to support proteomics studies. In addition, **Figure 2** provides a short list of the most promising and relevant salivary biomarkers discussed to date.

Acknowledgements

The authors thank the Portuguese Foundation for Science and Technology (FCT), European Union, QREN, FEDER and COMPETE for funding UnIC - Unidade de Investigação Cardiovascular (UIDB/00051/2020 and UIDP/00051/2020), iBiMED (UIDB/04501/2020, POCI-01-0145-FEDER-007628) and FCT LAQV/REQUIMTE (UIDB/50006/2020) research units. R.V. is supported by individual fellowship grants (IF/00286/2015). This work is funded by national funds (OE), through FCT Fundação para a Ciência e a Tecnologia , I.P., in the scope of the framework contract foreseen in the numbers 4, 5 and 6 of the article 23, of the Decree-Law 57/2016, of August 29, changed by Law 57/2017, of July 19.

Conflicts of interest

The authors declare no conflicts of interest.

Author details

Luís Perpétuo[1], Rita Ferreira[2], Sofia Guedes[2], Francisco Amado[2]
and Rui Vitorino[1,2,3]*

1 iBiMED, Department of Medical Sciences, University of Aveiro, Aveiro

2 LAQV/REQUIMTE, Department of Chemistry, University of Aveiro, Aveiro

3 Departamento de Cirurgia e Fisiologia, Faculdade de Medicina da Universidade do Porto, UnIC, Porto

*Address all correspondence to: rvitorino@ua.pt

References

[1] Khurshid Z, Zohaib S, Najeeb S, Zafar MS, Slowey PD, Almas K. Human saliva collection devices for proteomics: an update. International journal of molecular sciences, 17(6), 846 (2016).

[2] Dawes C. Salivary flow patterns and the health of hard and soft oral tissues. The Journal of the American Dental Association, 139, 18S-24S (2008).

[3] Podzimek S, Vondrackova L, Duskova J, Janatova T, Broukal Z. Salivary markers for periodontal and general diseases. Disease markers, 2016 (2016).

[4] Khurshid Z, Zafar MS, Khan RS, Najeeb S, Slowey PD, Rehman IU. Role of salivary biomarkers in oral cancer detection. Advances in clinical chemistry, 86, 23-70 (2018).

[5] Abdul Rehman S, Khurshid Z, Hussain Niazi F et al. Role of salivary biomarkers in detection of cardiovascular diseases (CVD). Proteomes, 5(3), 21 (2017).

[6] Saitou M, Gaylord E, Xu E et al. Functional specialization of human salivary glands and origins of proteins intrinsic to human saliva. bioRxiv, 2020.2002.2012.945659 (2020).

[7] Feizi A, Gatto F, Uhlen M, Nielsen J. Human protein secretory pathway genes are expressed in a tissue-specific pattern to match processing demands of the secretome. npj Systems Biology and Applications, 3(1), 22 (2017).

[8] Chansaenroj A, Yodmuang S, Ferreira JN. Trends in salivary gland tissue engineering: from stem cells to secretome and organoid bioprinting. Tissue Engineering Part B: Reviews, (2020).

[9] Hassaneen M, Maron JL. Salivary diagnostics in pediatrics: applicability, translatability, and limitations. Frontiers in public health, 5, 83 (2017).

[10] Pappa E, Kousvelari E, Vastardis H. Saliva in the "Omics" era: A promising tool in paediatrics. Oral diseases, 25(1), 16-25 (2019).

[11] Khurshid Z, Zohaib S, Najeeb S, Zafar MS, Rehman R, Rehman IU. Advances of proteomic sciences in dentistry. International journal of molecular sciences, 17(5), 728 (2016).

[12] Rahim MAA, Rahim ZHA, Ahmad WAW, Hashim OH. Can saliva proteins be used to predict the onset of acute myocardial infarction among high-risk patients? International journal of medical sciences, 12(4), 329 (2015).

[13] Wang X, Kaczor-Urbanowicz KE, Wong DT. Salivary biomarkers in cancer detection. Medical Oncology, 34(1), 1-8 (2017).

[14] Roi A, Rusu LC, Roi CI, Luca RE, Boia S, Munteanu RI. A new approach for the diagnosis of systemic and oral diseases based on salivary biomolecules. Disease markers, 2019 (2019).

[15] Meinken J, Walker G, Cooper CR, Min XJ. MetazSecKB: the human and animal secretome and subcellular proteome knowledgebase. Database, 2015 (2015).

[16] Silberring J, Ciborowski P. Biomarker discovery and clinical proteomics. TrAC Trends in Analytical Chemistry, 29(2), 128-140 (2010).

[17] Wang A, Wang CP, Tu M, Wong DT. Oral biofluid biomarker research: current

status and emerging frontiers. Diagnostics, 6(4), 45 (2016).

[18] Hsu C-W, Yu J-S, Peng P-H et al. Secretome profiling of primary cells reveals that THBS2 is a salivary biomarker of oral cavity squamous cell carcinoma. Journal of proteome research, 13(11), 4796-4807 (2014).

[19] Wei F, Wong D. Point-of-care platforms for salivary diagnostics. The Chinese journal of dental research: the official journal of the Scientific Section of the Chinese Stomatological Association (CSA), 15(1), 7-15 (2012).

[20] Soper SA, Brown K, Ellington A et al. Point-of-care biosensor systems for cancer diagnostics/prognostics. Biosensors and Bioelectronics, 21(10), 1932-1942 (2006).

[21] McRae MP, Simmons GW, Wong J et al. Programmable bio-nano-chip system: a flexible point-of-care platform for bioscience and clinical measurements. Lab on a Chip, 15(20), 4020-4031 (2015).

[22] Ngounou Wetie AG, Sokolowska I, Woods AG et al. Automated mass spectrometry–based functional assay for the routine analysis of the secretome. Journal of laboratory automation, 18(1), 19-29 (2013).

[23] Hosseini S, Espinosa-Hernandez MA, Garcia-Ramirez R, Cerda-Kipper AS, Reveles-Huizar S, Acosta-Soto L. BioMEMS.).

[24] Espinosa-Hernandez MA, Reveles-Huizar S, Hosseini S. Bio-microelectromechanical Systems (BioMEMS) in Bio-sensing Applications-Colorimetric Detection Strategies. In: BioMEMS. (Springer, 2021) 21-67.

[25] Naher S, Orpen D, Brabazon D, Morshed MM. An overview of microfluidic mixing application. In: Advanced Materials Research. (Ed.^(Eds) (Trans Tech Publ, 2010) 931-939.

[26] Morris MC. Fluorescent biosensors—probing protein kinase function in cancer and drug discovery. Biochimica et Biophysica Acta (BBA)-Proteins and Proteomics, 1834(7), 1387-1395 (2013).

[27] Mitchell AC, Alford SC, Hunter SA et al. Development of a protease biosensor based on a dimerization-dependent red fluorescent protein. ACS chemical biology, 13(1), 66-72 (2018).

[28] Tu M, Cheng J, Chen Y-L et al. Electric Field–Induced Release and Measurement (EFIRM): Characterization and Technical Validation of a Novel Liquid Biopsy Platform in Plasma and Saliva. The Journal of Molecular Diagnostics, 22(8), 1050-1062 (2020).

[29] Wei F, Strom CM, Cheng J et al. Electric field–induced release and measurement liquid biopsy for noninvasive early lung cancer assessment. The Journal of Molecular Diagnostics, 20(6), 738-742 (2018).

[30] Mani V, Beduk T, Khushaim W et al. Electrochemical sensors targeting salivary biomarkers: A comprehensive review. TrAC Trends in Analytical Chemistry, 116164 (2020).

[31] Goswami Y, Mishra R, Agrawal AP, Agrawal LA. Salivary biomarkers: A review of powerful diagnostic tool. IOSR J. Dental Med. Sci, 14(3), 80-87 (2015).

[32] Yoshizawa JM, Schafer CA, Schafer JJ, Farrell JJ, Paster BJ, Wong DT. Salivary biomarkers: toward future clinical and diagnostic utilities. Clinical microbiology reviews, 26(4), 781-791 (2013).

[33] Gug IT, Tertis M, Hosu O, Cristea C. Salivary biomarkers detection: Analytical and immunological methods overview. TrAC Trends in Analytical Chemistry, 113, 301-316 (2019).

[34] Castagnola M, Scarano E, Passali G et al. Salivary biomarkers and proteomics: future diagnostic and clinical utilities. Acta Otorhinolaryngologica Italica, 37(2), 94 (2017).

[35] Sivadasan P, Gupta MK, Sathe GJ et al. Data from human salivary proteome–A resource of potential biomarkers for oral cancer. Data in brief, 4, 374-378 (2015).

[36] Proctor GB. The physiology of salivary secretion. Periodontology 2000, 70(1), 11-25 (2016).

[37] Keremi B, Beck A, Karoly Fabian T et al. Stress and salivary glands. Current pharmaceutical design, 23(27), 4057-4065 (2017).

[38] Wang J, Liang Y, Wang Y et al. Computational prediction of human salivary proteins from blood circulation and application to diagnostic biomarker identification. PLoS One, 8(11), e80211 (2013).

[39] Caccia D, Dugo M, Callari M, Bongarzone I. Bioinformatics tools for secretome analysis. Biochimica et Biophysica Acta (BBA)-Proteins and Proteomics, 1834(11), 2442-2453 (2013).

[40] Ashburner M, Ball CA, Blake JA et al. Gene ontology: tool for the unification of biology. Nature genetics, 25(1), 25-29 (2000).

[41] Khatri P, Drăghici S. Ontological analysis of gene expression data: current tools, limitations, and open problems. Bioinformatics, 21(18), 3587-3595 (2005).

[42] Szklarczyk D, Franceschini A, Kuhn M et al. The STRING database in 2011: functional interaction networks of proteins, globally integrated and scored. Nucleic acids research, 39(suppl_1), D561-D568 (2010).

[43] Cline MS, Smoot M, Cerami E et al. Integration of biological networks and gene expression data using Cytoscape. Nature protocols, 2(10), 2366 (2007).

[44] Ma Z-Q, Tabb DL, Burden J et al. Supporting tool suite for production proteomics. Bioinformatics, 27(22), 3214-3215 (2011).

[45] Martens L, Chambers M, Sturm M et al. mzML—a community standard for mass spectrometry data. Molecular & Cellular Proteomics, 10(1), R110. 000133 (2011).

[46] Orchard S, Hermjakob H. The HUPO proteomics standards initiative—easing communication and minimizing data loss in a changing world. Briefings in bioinformatics, 9(2), 166-173 (2008).

[47] Deutsch EW, Lam H, Aebersold R. PeptideAtlas: a resource for target selection for emerging targeted proteomics workflows. EMBO reports, 9(5), 429-434 (2008).

[48] Jones P, Martens L. Using the PRIDE proteomics identifications database for knowledge discovery and data analysis. In: Proteome Bioinformatics. (Springer, 2010) 297-307.

[49] Smith BE, Hill JA, Gjukich MA, Andrews PC. Tranche distributed repository and ProteomeCommons. org. In: Data Mining in Proteomics. (Springer, 2011) 123-145.

[50] Rehman AU, Olof Olsson P, Khan N, Khan K. Identification of Human Secretome and Membrane

Proteome-Based Cancer Biomarkers Utilizing Bioinformatics. The Journal of membrane biology, 253, 257-270 (2020).

[51] Shin J, Rhim J, Kwon Y et al. Comparative analysis of differentially secreted proteins in serum-free and serum-containing media by using BONCAT and pulsed SILAC. Scientific reports, 9(1), 1-12 (2019).

[52] Min XJ. Evaluation of computational methods for secreted protein prediction in different eukaryotes. JPB, 3(5) (2010).

[53] Uhlén M, Fagerberg L, Hallström BM et al. Tissue-based map of the human proteome. Science, 347(6220) (2015).

[54] Keerthikumar S. A catalogue of human secreted proteins and its implications. AIMS Biophys, 3(4), 563-570 (2016).

[55] Chen G, Chen J, Liu H et al. Comprehensive identification and characterization of human secretome based on integrative proteomic and transcriptomic data. Frontiers in cell and developmental biology, 7, 299 (2019).

[56] Mona M, Kobeissy F, Park Y-J et al. Secretome Analysis of Inductive Signals for BM-MSC Transdifferentiation into Salivary Gland Progenitors. International journal of molecular sciences, 21(23), 9055 (2020).

[57] Khan RS, Khurshid Z, Yahya Ibrahim Asiri F. Advancing point-of-care (PoC) testing using human saliva as liquid biopsy. Diagnostics, 7(3), 39 (2017).

Chapter 2

Endothelial Secretome

Luiza Rusu

Abstract

Endothelial cells produce huge proteomes from a relatively small total number of ECs. The ECs' complex intercellular communication is possible through well-stored, classified, and compartmentalized secretory pathways, intermediated by the secretory vesicles and granules, with the purpose to maintain vascular homeostasis and integrity. Secreted proteins are involved in a myriad of cell communication processes. The local vascular microenvironment dynamically and constantly modifies the ECs' secretome. We focus on the biological significance of secretome proteins in a healthy vascular microenvironment and under cardiovascular conditions. Vascular ECs crosstalk with other ECs, and other blood cells at a distance, with the circulating hematopoietic stem cells permitting adequate reactions to vascular injury, systemic or local inflammation, and viral or parasitic infections. Here, we overview current secretome biomarkers in vascular diseases, with a focus on their roles in diagnostic, prognostic, and therapeutics. Also, we highlighted some important pathological effects of exosome on cardiovascular disease. This chapter discusses current research directions characterizing vascular pathology conditioned secretomes, their regulation, and therapeutic pursuit. The overall aim of this chapter is to review current literature updates on endothelial secretome roles in endothelial homeostasis and in vascular disorders.

Keywords: endothelial cells, secretome, Weibel–Palade bodies, extracellular vesicles, exosomes, signal transduction, intercellular crosstalk, secretory pathways, ectodomain shedding

1. Introduction

Endothelium consists of approximately 10^{14} cells in all the vasculature [1]. Due to its versatile functions, the endothelium has been compared with a metabolic organ [1]. The ECs' secretomes comprise all proteins secreted outside the cell, including enzymes, growth factors, and hormones. ECs have the most diverse regulatory roles, starting with a mechanical barrier, vascular tone, hemostasis, and thrombosis (including control of platelet response), inflammation, vascular permeability, and angiogenesis. The interactions of ECs with leukocytes are also mediated by constituents of the ECs' secretome. The local microenvironment influences ECs' secretome output. For instance, the presence or absence of certain constituents in the secretory vesicles or granules can be selectively changed by local inflammation or by shear stress [2]. Endothelial cells produce huge proteomes from a relatively small total number of ECs. This is possible by well-stored, classified, and compartmentalized polarized exocytosis [3]. Exchange information at a distance with other ECs, and with other blood cells, with the circulating hematopoietic stem cells. Vascular ECs crosstalk is intermediated by the secretory vesicles and granules with the purpose to maintain vascular homeostasis and integrity [4].

Despite the crucial role endothelial secretome is playing in EC function, we are only recently started to understand the molecular mechanisms governing the EC secretory function. In 2009, the first proteomic analysis on cultured HUVEC was conducted, and that study identified a number of 374 secreted proteins using nanoflow LC–MS/MS permitting the identification of angiogenic factors, extracellular matrix components, proteins involved in coagulation and inflammation, and in vascular tone, permeability and regeneration, and atherosclerosis and dissemination of metastasis [3]. More recently, 183 proteins were identified to be associated with the main secretory granules in quiescent HUVECS by proximity proteomics [5]. Meanwhile, a lot of progress was made in these regards, while some aspects are still under elucidation.

ECs intercellular crosstalk, which is mostly happening in the extracellular space, is highly controlled by ECs secretory pathways. It implies a donor (parent) cell which packs its contents into vesicles and a target (acceptor) cell that internalizes and uptake the vesicles. Endothelial cell secretory pathways occur via different size vesicles as follows: exocytosis of the principal secretory granules, Weibel–Palade bodies, and through smaller secretory granules, extracellular vesicles, and exosomes. Shedding of the ectodomain also provides many receptors and ligands for the target (recipient or acceptor) cell [6].

The main secretory storage granules of the ECs are Weibel–Palade bodies (WPBs), which represent the bulk source of stored, highly multimeric von Willebrand factor (vWF) [7]. The only other sources of vWF in the body are megakaryocytes and platelets α-granules, but they provide vWF in much smaller quantities only when stimulated [8]. WPBs are highly specialized organelles that ensure that ECs can promptly, and time-dependently respond to vascular injury or stress by enabling the controlled release of hemostasis and angiogenic factors, like vWF and not only to maintain vascular integrity. WPBs are large storage granules, their size ranges between 1 and 5 μm long and 100–300 nm wide, therefore, they are ideal for microscopy studies for secretion visualization from vascular endothelial cells.

Recent studies provide novel insights regarding endothelial secretome. Importantly, a recently published ***proximity proteomics study*** from Holthenrich et al. [5] provided interesting updates regarding ***WPB secretion regulation factors and the endothelial secretome***.

EVs were first described in Peter Wolf as "platelet dust" and first characterized in 2011 by Gyorgy et al. [9] EVs are complex vesicular structures responsible for intercellular communication by transferring between cells: cytosolic proteins (e.g., enzymes and cytoskeletal proteins), lipids, mRNA, miRNA, and organelles from the parent cell.

EVs are released by virtually all cell types. EVs were identified in most body fluids and in the tissue matrix [10, 11]. Vesicles distinguish from one another based on size and density range and the mechanisms leading to their formation [12]. EVs originating from the cell membrane, by exposing to the exterior of the cytosolic side, by outward blebbing and budding, are named ***microvesicles, ectosomes,*** or ***microparticles*** [13, 14]. EVs that originate from the intracellular endocytic trafficking pathway is budding inward from the endosomal compartment, accumulate in multivesicular bodies (MVBs) in the form of many intraluminal vesicles [13] that upon fusion of the limiting membrane of MVBs with the plasma membrane, are released as ***exosomes*** [9, 14, 15]. EC-derived EVs biogenesis is lipid rafts-dependent and ADP-ribosylation factor 6 (ARF6)-dependent [16].

Several regulator molecules localized simultaneously on the EVs surface, and on the EC acceptor cells are known to be implicated in the delivery of cargo and uptake into the target cell, including integrins and integrin-associated proteins, tetraspanins, T-cell immunoglobulin, and mucin domain-containing protein-4 (TIM4), and lectins and heparan sulfate proteoglycans [4]. Tim4 is a receptor for TIM1 and phosphatidylserine on apoptotic cells. Without Tim4, macrophages cannot phagocytose apoptotic cells. These molecular pairs convey cargo delivery specifically to the vascular recipient cells, although it is not entirely clear how these processes occur [4].

EVs transfer their cargo from the parent cell to the target cell by: (1) docking to the target cell, (2) internalization of the EVs, and intracellular sorting through one of the endocytotic pathways; a pool of internalized EVs by the acceptor (target) cells are sent via endosomal escape, and (3) transfer of the EV content to the acceptor cell [4]. This way EVs influence the phenotypic traits of the recipient cell. Importantly, the released exosomes conserve many transmembrane proteins from the parent ECs.

ECs release into the extracellular space diverse types of EC-derived lipid membranal bilayer-enclosed structures in response to cellular activation or apoptosis, these microparticles have ambivalent functions (both favorable and detrimental) in vascular homeostasis.

In all, the aim of this chapter is to review current literature updates on endothelial secretome's roles in endothelial homeostasis and in vascular disorders. We focus on the biological significance of secretome proteins in the vascular microenvironment in health and under different cardiovascular conditions. Secretome biomarkers in vascular diseases will be overviewed, with a focus on their roles in diagnostic, prognostic, and therapeutics. We highlight the important pathological effects of exosomes in cardiovascular disease. Most importantly, this chapter discusses vascular pathology conditioned secretomes, their regulation, and future therapeutic pursuit.

2. EC Secretome and exocytosis

2.1 Weibel: palade bodies (WPBs)–History, biogenesis, mechanisms, and pathogenesis

Discovery of WPBs - Edward Weibel and George Emil Palade were the first to describe WPBs in the early sixties by examining small arteries with a transmission electron microscope as "a hitherto unknown rod-shaped cytoplasmic component which consists of a bundle of fine tubules, enveloped by a tightly fitted membrane, was regularly found in endothelial cells of small arteries in various organs in rat and man." [17] In TEM transversal section, WPBs are electrono-dense tubules packed in parallel bundles encapsulated in a lipid membrane. The tubules inside WPBs have a diameter of circa 12 nm and appear to be surrounded by a dense matrix, and sometimes they have a hinge at the end of the organelle. After WPBs discovery, it took approximately 20 years until the discovery of the main WPBs components. WPBs is the best example of a secretory organelle whose formation is dictated by vWF, its main storage constituent. vWF is secreted in the form of ultra-large multimers in response to the multitude of stimuli that activate ECs. vWF-deficient mice do not form EC WPBs [18]. Reversely, overexpression of vWF in other cell types leads to the formation of WPB-like granules with similar morphology: rod-shaped and striated granules [19, 20].

WPBs biogenesis - vWF is synthesized in the rough endoplasmic reticulum as a sequence of precursor conserved domains, as follows: D1-D2-D′-D3-A1-A2-A3-D4-B1-B2-B3-C1-C2-CK [21]. Consequently, furin, a pH-dependent enzyme, cleaves down the D1-D2 domain (approximately 100 kDa and ~ 750 aa) during the trans-Golgi network (TGN) processing step [21]. The sequence starting from the domain D′ and up to the cysteine knot (CK) domain represents the mature vWF [21, 22]. As vWF passes through the Golgi complex, it suffers more processing. At the level of the TGN, the presence of vWF leads to the biogenesis of WPBs [21]. In the TGN, vWF dimers go through the process of multimerization by bridging the D3 domains via interchain N-terminal disulfide bonds [22, 23]. In the TGN, WPBs go through a process of maturation and are directed, when needed, toward the basolateral surface in small vesicles [24] or stored in the highly multimerized form in WPBs [24] for later use via regulated secretion [21]. WPBs that protrude from the TGN have clathrin/AP1 coats on [25]. Overexpression of the dominant-negative construct AP180 and AP-1 inhibition with siRNA inhibits the formation of the clathrin coat. Therefore, it is considered that clathrin/AP1 are essential in the formation of vWF tubules and for their correct packaging [25]. Aftiphilin and y-synergin are the downstream effectors of AP-1, which are recruited to the WPBs, as shown by their fluorescence microscopical partial colocalization with immature WPBs situated perinuclearly. Their depletion with siRNA does not modify the total number of WPBs or their intracellular distribution, but it increased the basal secretion of vWF and reduces the regulated vWF secretion [26]. vWF propeptide is necessary for WPBs biogenesis [20]. The vWF tubules are only forming at the level of TGN, not before, in the Golgi complex [25]. Immature (perinuclear) WPBs have different membrane protein sets than mature (cytoplasmic) WPBs. Upon maturation of WPBs, they lose their clathrin/AP-1 coat and its effectors aftiphilin and synergin [25, 26]. The tetraspanin CD63 is recruited to the mature WPBs with the help of the adaptor AP3, which targets proteins from endosome to the lysosome and related organelles. Lysosomal organelles, such as melanosomes and α-granules, have the characteristic to sort endosomal proteins into secretory granules after Golgi processing [27]. After the processing and maturation process, WPBs can be stored in the ECs for long times, for a few days [28].

WPBs exocytosis - vWF released from WPBs of vascular ECs has a crucial function in hemostasis and thrombosis. Under physiological conditions, WPBs have a low rate of basal secretion into the bloodstream that is thought to be required to maintain the blood level of VWF. The blood level of vWF is thought to be originating from the ECs exclusively, while the platelet α-granules and readily formed WPBs can supplement vWF released upon platelet activation. Under stimulation, the rate of WPBs can be rapidly increased by Ca^{2+}- or by a cAMP-induced secretory mechanism. Upon activation of ECs, highly multimeric vWF is liberated from WPBs through the apical side of EC toward the bloodstream. Activated ECs lead to the regulated exocytosis of WPBs. As vWF is liberated from WPBs, it unfurls into long (1–5 μm) “strings” that platelets recognize via the A1 domain of vWF as “beads on the string” to initiate platelet adhesion and aggregation and the formation of a thrombus plug. Moreover, it vehiculated the idea that the contents of WPBs can be specifically altered, depending on where in the vasculature bed of which organs are ECs located. Ca^{2+} and cAMP-dependent controlled WPBs exocytosis regulate the local vascular environment to mediate the interconnected processes of hemostasis, vascular inflammation, and thrombosis. The molecular mechanisms controlling the trafficking of ECs secretory granules were only partially elucidated. We know that WPB priming and exocytosis are mediated by the N-ethylmaleimide factor, α-SNARE adaptor protein (α-SNAP), and SNARE receptors. WPB exocytosis depends on syntaxin 4, members of the SNARE complexes, synaptobrevin 3, synaptotagmin, and a sensor for Ca2 + −mediated exocytosis. In addition, nitric oxide (NO) was found to influence negatively NSF function by S-nitrosylation and inhibiting ECs exocytosis of vWF [29].

In addition, Weibel–Palade bodies contain P-selectin, other selectins, Rab27a, endothelin-1, endothelin-converting enzyme, angiopoietin, CD63, tissue-type plasminogen activator (tPA), interleukins (IL) IL-1, IL-8, CCL-2, eotaxin-3, osteoprotegerin, and calcitonin-gene related protein [30]. The question of cytokines incorporation into WPBs was recently revisited, Il1 and IL8 were found in WPBs but other cytokines are transported via other vesicles. These other components of WPBs like P-selectin, cytokines, and osteoprotegerin are incorporated during the processing phase in the TGN. P-selectin is a transmembranar protein, which is highly relevant for leukocyte rolling. Its big luminal domain is sufficient for the incorporation of P-selectin into the WPBs, even if truncated, probably because of its interaction with D′ and D3 domains of vWF [31, 32]. P-selectin is produced and stored in WPBs and the α-granules of platelets. P-selectin affects the formation of WPBs, andthe recruitment of leukocytes in vWF-deficient animals [33, 34].

The secretome of WPBs is characterized by dynamics and plasticity to meet the versatility of ECs pathophysiology [30]. Clotting factor VIII is stored in pulmonary ECs in association with vWF [35]. Osteoprotegerin is also stored in WPBs and its incorporation in WPBs is related to its interaction with vWF [7]. Osteoprotegerin (OPG) is one of the tumor necrosis factors (TNF) cytokine receptors [36]. Osteoprotegerin is involved in the inhibition of bone regeneration via OPG/the receptor activator of nuclear factor kappa-B (RANK)/receptor activator of nuclear factor kappa-B ligand (RANKL) axis, by decreasing the production of osteoclasts [36]. Another study focused on WPB resident proteins identified IGFBP7 by proteomic screening [7]. Angiopoietin-2 is part of a family of four growth factors whose activity is mediated via tyrosine kinase receptors (Tie) receptors 1 and 2. Angiopoietin-2 has different functions depending on the microenvironment conditions, an autocrine regulator, and an antagonist of Tie2. In activated ECs, vascular endothelial growth factor (VEGF) stimulation of angiopoietin-2 has proinflammatory effects. Angiopoietin-2 is incorporated into WPBs, at the level of TGN, if there is no P-selectin present because these two factors are mutually exclusive [37]. Angiopoietin-2 expression is induced by local inflammatory and prothrombotic factors, such as thrombin or under hypoxic conditions, and its release is highly regulated.

A recent study employed a new approach involving **proximity proteomics** to find proteins residing on the cytosolic face of the WPBs or in the vicinity of the organelle. In this case, biotinylating the target proteins in living cultured HUVECs followed by streptavidin pulldown and identification of the new proteins by tandem mass spectrometry [5]. The small GTPases Rab3b and Rab27 were previously identified in the proximity of WPBs on the cytoplasmic face of WPBs. In this study, the authors show that the two mentioned Rab small GTPases fused with peroxidase APEX2, and modified ascorbate peroxidase [5]. In this study, HUVECs were transfected with Rab3b tagged with FLAG-APEX2 construct. The resulted proteins were immunoblotted with anti-FLAG antibodies. Proteins associated with WPBs that were tagged, and upon adding biotin-phenol and peroxide of hydrogen for 1 minute there was peroxidase-catalyzed biotinylation of the protein in the vicinity of WPBs as shown by streptavidin pulldown from the pretreated HUVECs under resting conditions. The pulldowns were sent to tandem mass spectrometry.

This approach led to the identification of a total number of 183 proteins associated with WPBs and with one of the two Rab GTPases or with both constructs. Many of those were not identified in the vicinity or in association with WPB before. Importantly, these proteins were previously found to be related to membrane/protein transport or to organelle dynamics and plasticity. Vacuolar ATPase ATP6V, syntaxin binding protein 1, Rab 46, phospholipase D1, GBF1, and phosphatidylinositol 4-kinase were identified as WPBs constituents, some of them were previously known to be related to WPBs exocytosis [5]. Rab 7, one of the proteins identified by proximity proteomics was thought to regulate the transport from endosome to WPBs [5]. Some Golgin family members were also identified by the same approach. The secretory pathway Ca^{2+} ATPase type 1 is another newly discovered constituent of WPBs, which is known to be involved in Ca^{2+} homeostasis [5]. The fact that well-known markers of WPBs, such as P-selectin, VAMP-3, CD63, MyRIP, and Slp4a, were recognized in this study verifies the specificity of their approach. A previous study showed that the interplay between Rab27A and its effectors Slp-4 and MyRIP controls histamine-induced vWF secretion [38]. CD63 is well known to be associated with WPBs.

Importantly, one new protein associated with WPBs by proximity ligation is the priming/tethering factor Munc 13-2, which is a positive regulator of histamine-induced WPB exocytosis of vWF [5]. Munc 13-2 was previously implicated in WPB exocytosis of angiopoietin-2 from the brain ECs [39]. After the initial proteomic screening and verification, Munc 13-2 localizes at WPB surface, and they also demonstrated that Munc 13-2 siRNA affects histamine-induced vWF secretion [5]. In addition, Munc 13-2 cooperates with Munc 13-4, which was found to be a plasma membrane priming and fusion factor for evoked WPBs exocytosis [5].

WPBs defects - Defects in the structure, packing, or sorting of vWF lead to von Willebrand disease (vWD), which has an incidence of approximately 1:1000 in general population and represents the most common inherited coagulopathy in humans. The inherited defects in vWF result in smaller and defective WPBs. Defects in the proteins that regulate WPB exocytosis also led to vWD. Reversely, excess of vWF released by activated ECs exposed to high shear stress or to vascular inflammation, or infection tilts the thrombotic propensity leading to disseminated intravascular coagulation and microvascular thrombosis.

2.2 Secretory granules, vesicles of 100–500 nm diameter which store cargo of smaller dimensions

The initial belief that cytokines reside exclusively in WPBs in vascular ECs from where they are released upon stimulation, that is, with histamine, was recently challenged [40]. The question of cytokines incorporation into WPBs was recently revisited, Il-1 and IL-8 were found in WPBs but other cytokines are transported via other vesicles. It was proven that cytokines originate and are also secreted from smaller vesicles by vascular ECs and that cytokines (monocyte-chemoattractant protein-1 [MCP-1], IL-6, and IL-8), EGFP, and tissue plasminogen (tPA) are much less efficiently stored in WPBs compared with vWF, but are present in "tPA and type 2 organelles." [40] Chemokines are small cytokines that direct the movement of cells during embryogenesis, in order to maintain homeostasis or in pathological conditions. Their roles include cell proliferation, cell migration, cell differentiation, and implicit maintaining tissue and organs homeostasis by regulating the types and number of each cell produced. ECs express cytokines, such as interleukins (IL) IL-1, IL-5, IL-6, IL-8, IL-11, and IL-15, granulocyte/macrophage colony-stimulating factor (GM-CSF). Upon local or systemic vascular inflammation, secretion of a particular set of cytokines can attract specifically certain subtypes of leukocytes. ECs secrete chemokines, such as CCL2 (attracts monocytes), CCL5 (monocytes, eosinophils, and T cells), eotaxin-3/CCL26 (eosinophils), CXCL1 (to attract neutrophils), and CXCL10 (for T cells) [41–43]. Activated ECs secrete upon vascular injury by other coagulation agents, such as plasminogen activator inhibitor-1 (PAI-1) or other growth hormones like TGF-β [42].

Much of the intercellular communication performed by vascular ECs is done by means of soluble cytokines and chemokines. Upon endothelial cell activation during inflammation, cytokines are released from EC secretory vesicles, and there is vasodilation to lower the blood flow and recruitment of leukocytes at the site of infection or injury. The first step is the vasodilation of the blood vessel, which allows for better leukocytes interaction with the vascular ECs. Vasodilatation is partly a result of EC-induced mechanisms. The endothelium secretes increased the level of P- and E-selectins, intracellular adhesion molecules (ICAM), and integrins. 1) **rolling adhesion**: The initial low-affinity endothelial-leukocyte interactions involve an increased level of selectins. P-selectin is secreted from WPBs in minutes, in response to histamine released by mast cells or mediated by TNF-α or LPS. TNF-α is one type of molecule produced by macrophages in response to pathogen detection, causing endothelial activation. Histamine-mediated activated ECs rapidly externalize WPBs content, which includes preformed P-selectin. TNF-α or LPS induce the synthesis of E-selectin, which is exposed to the cell surface a few hours later. Selectins recognize Sialyl-LewisX on the rolling leukocytes across the endothelium, allowing them to adhere reversibly (tethering or capture) to the vascular wall. Without these initial interactions, the next steps of chemokine-dependent and chemokine-independent mechanisms leukocyte activation, and extravasation would not occur. These steps depend on the production and adequate release of P-selectins from WPB granules of vascular ECs. 2) **Leukocyte-Endothelial tight binding** relies on integrins (VLA-4, CD18, and CD11) on leukocytes and ICAMs on the surface of vascular ECs, such as TNF-α-induced endothelial ICAM-1, or ICAM-2, and VCAM-1 3, **diapedesis** is the step in which the leukocyte extravasate the endothelial wall. This step involves the interaction of integrins (CD11/CD18 and VLA-4) on leukocytes with ICAMs on ECs (i.e., ICAM-1 and VCAM-1), and with PECAM-1 (CD31).

2.3 Secretome trafficking via extracellular vesicles (EVs)

2.3.1 Secretome trafficking via endothelial microvesicles (MVs)

Endothelial MVs are plasma membrane-derived vesicles, they occur through blebbing and budding of the cell membrane starting intracellularly from the cytosol, budding toward the exterior of the cell [12]. Their size ranges from 100 to 2000 nm [15]. The majority of MVs come from platelets. Vesicles should be collected from plasma not from serum because activation of platelets leads to excessive release of platelets MVs, and contamination of the sample.

EVs reflect the status of the patent cell. EC-derived EVs can be released with the purpose to protect the endothelium from distress, therefore, they fulfill the function of gatekeepers, with cytoprotective and antiapoptotic effects.

One of the factors known to regulate the biogenesis of the microparticles is ARF6 [16].

EC-derived MVs carry markers/regulator proteins that are associated with a pathological state: vascular endothelial cadherin (VE-cadherin), endoglin (CD105), (c-Src kinase+, eNOS+ and caveolin1+, EPCR+). ECs-derived MVs from plasma of septic mice had increased levels of VE-cadherin+ and endoglin+ vesicles compared to sham control. EC-derived MVs applied *in vitro* on cultured ECs cause endothelial permeability dysfunctions by disturbing the adherens junctions and the cytoskeleton [44]. Platelet endothelial cell adhesion molecule-1 (CD31+ or PECAM-1), E-selectin, αv integrin (CD51), and intercellular cell adhesion molecule (ICAM)-1 (cytokine-stimulated HUVECs released increased levels of both factors; moreover, E-selectin-targeting to inflamed ECs help delivery of miRNAs from MVs, with anti-inflammatory effects [45]), or S-endo (CD146) [45], endothelial NO synthase, oxidated negatively charged phospholipids (infusion with man-made negatively charged phospholipid vesicles leads to severe thrombosis in primates and murine models [46]), and vascular endothelial growth factor receptor (VEGF-R2) [47]. High adhesion molecules level constitute a sign of endothelial dysfunction and decreased vessel elasticity [46].

Because the presence of EVs released by ECs in the circulation usually indicates a vascular or systemic disease, they can be used as markers of endothelial dysfunction. The endothelial origin of circulating MVs can be established by flow cytometry and other laboratory tests. One caveat is that, apart from E-selectin and VE-cadherin, these protein markers are not expressed exclusively by the vascular cells.

In the case of transfer of membrane-bound MVs by cocultures, recipient cells take some phenotypic characteristics of the MV-producing cells; sick or degenerative cell regain their normal phenotype, and a bidirectional membrane transfer is observed between cells. Circulating EVs can be distinguished by tissue source and disease state profiling. EVs are molecular heterogeneous and overlap a lot. There is also large heterogeneity in the mechanical properties of EVs that may dictate cellular behavior.

2.3.2 Secretome trafficking through exosomes

Exosomes are nanoscale vesicles with a diameter ranging between 30 and 150 nm. Exosomes can be released from any type of cell in the body, their release is higher from certain cell types. Exosomes originate from the intracellular endocytic trafficking pathway, during the endosome compartment maturation in MVBs; MVBs membrane fusion with the cell membrane allows the release of their intraluminal vesicle as exosomes, as shown by electron microscopic shots of exosomes that previously endocytosed colloidal gold [15].

Exosome biogenesis involves a two-step budding process: step 1) inward budding of the external plasma membrane through the endocytotic pathway to the endosomal compartment and intraluminal vesicles into MVBs and step 2) cytosolic MVBs secrete the exosome cargo. Importantly, the released exosomes conserve many transmembrane proteins from the parent ECs.

Silencing the endosomal sorting complex transport protein (ESCRT) members, ESCRT-0 and/or ESCRT-I, decreases exosome secretion [48], and modified the size of exosomes and their composition, and major histocompatibility complexes (MHC) levels, especially, impaired MHC II content, as shown by immunogold electron microscopy [48].

Several proteins are involved in exosome cargo sorting. Small GTPases Rab7a and Rab27b, found mainly on late endosomes, coordinate miRNA 143/miRNA150 export through nanovesicular trafficking, in response to the shear stress-inducible transcription factor Krüppel-like factor 2 (KLF2) overexpression, in cultured HUVECs, to levels that mimic shear stress levels [49]. The release of the exosome cargo goes through a Rab11- and Rab35-dependent regulatory pathway, which is involved in slow endocytic endosome recycling [49].

ShRNA knockdown of ESCRT-associated proteins, VTA, TSG101, VPS4, and ALG-2-interacting protein X increased exosome secretion, and increased MHC II proteic and mRNA content, as demonstrated on a 96-well plate screen of over 20 components of the ESCRT system and associated proteins [48].

Exosomes are characterized by: 1) expression of a set of integrins and tetraspanins (CD9, CD63, CD81, and CD82) for targeting and adhesion, 2) expression of proteins involved in membrane transport and fusion (annexins, Rab proteins, and flotillin), 3) expression of proteins associated with multivesicular body biogenesis (ALG-2-interacting protein X, TSG101, VPS4,a and VTA), 4) lipid-rafts (sphingolipids, sphingomyelinase, lipid ceramide, and cholesterol), 5) heat shock protein (HSP)-70 and – 90, as well as of 6) MHC I and II. 7) Another specific exosomal marker is a lysosomal-associated membrane protein-1 (Lamp1). 8) Importantly, EC-derived EVs contain miRNAs conveying immune responses.

Exosomes can be visualized on a NanoSight microscope. The uptake of endothelial exosomes, and the gain of function exosomes transfer can be measured.

Published data show that EC exosomes secreted in the circulation influence cellular behavior via paracrine signaling and can have huge biopotential: exosomes influence cell phenotypes, regulate protein synthesis, convey immune responses, stimulate angiogenesis, endothelial proliferation and migration, cell-free regeneration potential, and cardioprotective effects.

2.3.3 Caveolae

ECs also contain many caveolae, specialized endocytosis structures which are necessary for transcytosis of a variety of substances (i.e., albumin transport [5, 37] across the EC layer).

2.3.4 Tunneling nanotubules

Endothelial cells communicate with the help of tunneling nanotubes (TNT), which can be up to or more than 100 μm long and 50–200 nm in diameter. TNTs are composed of open-ended F-actin, nonadherent. TNTs form transiently for 30 minutes to 2 h and then retract and disappear.

2.4 Shedding of protein Ectodomains

Apart from the classical secretory pathways, about 2–4% of cell membrane proteins are released in circulation or into the extracellular space, in health or under pathological conditions, by ***ectodomain shedding,*** which is a proteolytic removal of a significant portion of the transmembrane protein ectodomain (the extracellular domain) [6]. Ectodomain shedding is relevant in growth factor signaling to cell adhesion, inflammation, cell survival, and cancer. The results of ectodomain shedding for ECs differ strongly depending on the type of shed transmembranar protein (i.e., adhesion molecules, growth factors, cytokines, and cell receptors). The shed enzymes are **membrane-bound proteolytic enzymes that cleave**, releasing the soluble ectodomains and leaving behind a protein fragment bound to the plasma membrane that can initiate signaling at this level or can be internalized in membrane-bound vesicles for unusual destination signaling in the nucleus to target gene activity or in the mitochondria.

ADAM17 and ADAM10 metalloproteases are the main sheddases expressed by ECs from the "a disintegrin and metalloprotease" (ADAM) family of sheddases. Upon inflammation, ADAM10 is responsible through a notch-dependent regulation for DII-1 and -4 expression and changes in Hes1 and Hey1 expression.

Among over 40 shedding substrates that ADAM10 has on resting and/or activated ECs, the most important ones include as follows: IL-6, Interleukin-6-receptor (IL-6R), IL-8 [50], CX3CL1, CD44, CXCL16, MCP-1, VEGFR2, sVCAM1 (on TNF-activated ECs) [51]. DLL4 and VE-cadherin (regulates endothelial permeability and transmigration [51–54].

2.5 Organotypic EC secretome

Location dictates the function; it was demonstrated over the years that the characteristics of the secretome of different subtypes of ECs are dependent on their localization in the vasculature bed. Distinct subtypes of ECS secrete tissue-specific proteomes, which regulate specifically tissue homeostasis and regeneration and functional pathophysiology. There are key features specific to the secretome of the continuous, discontinuous, fenestrated, sinusoidal, Schlemm's canal specialized ECs, and high endothelial venules. Brain, retina, and bones have organotypically differentiated ECs with specific morphological features that predict the functional particularities specific to the vessel bed and the tissue-specific EC secretome. Under physiological conditions, ECs have quiescent functions and phenotypic characteristics and they produce a different sets of vesicles and granules constituents upon activation. Quiescent ECs are not inactive though but under normal conditions they are inactive. They function as a gatekeeper in their microenvironment to control tissue function, homeostasis, and regeneration. As gatekeepers, ECs respond to different stimuli (inflammatory, infectious, metastasis, and high shear stress), they modify accordingly their phenotypes and functions to preserve vascular homeostasis. The molecular mechanisms controlling ECs vessel-bed specific differentiation and function are now emerging for protein preparation and secretion, and protein export into the extracellular microenvironment.

2.6 ECs apical and basolateral secretome

Endothelial cells have distinctive apical and basolateral secretomes. ECs polarize the secretion of small vesicles toward the apical side of ECs. For example, cytokines that are destined for blood circulation are secreted into the apical side of ECs. In contrast, the basolateral proteome is destined toward the components of the extracellular matrix, sharing their route with fibronectin and liprin-α1. The approach employed to dissect protein sorting in ECs to basolateral or apical compartments was to grow

HUVECs on transwell inserts with separate collecting compartments for basolateral and for the apical secretory pathways.

2.7 miRNAs transfer functionally using EVs

A microRNA is RNA that binds with imperfect complementarity to its target mRNA, might be 6–7 nucleotides long sequences, with a lot of opportunities for binding at the end of the target mRNA, and many non-canonical mechanisms were described so far. The difference between siRNA (which was described first) and miRNA is the degree of complementarity with the target. miRNA bind to its target leads to shutting down of translation by several mechanisms: translational inhibition, deadenylation, and cleavage in certain situations. At the heart of the miRNA mechanism is arg0naute protein (Ago), which is part of the miRNA-mediated gene silencing complex (RISC). miRNA is loaded with the argonaute as it is made, mature acts as part of argonaute RISC complex.

Rab GTPases regulate membrane trafficking for EC-derived vesicular miRNA [49]. In cultured ECs, the miR-143 vesicular export occurs through a Rab7a/Rab27b-dependent mechanism, induced by overexpression of the transcription factor KLF2 at levels that mimic high shear stress [49].

3. Role of endothelial Secretome in endothelial dysfunction

Dynamic vasculature regulation correlates (updates) ECs secretome with ECs functional needs in health, and under inflammatory conditions, under high shear stress, or under abnormal angiogenic factors.

Upon injury, cells are recruited by exosome-mediated receptor-mediated interactions, variety of responses occur in the vasculature because of the diverse mechanisms of action. Internalization of EC exosomes by monocytes/macrophages can suppress systemic inflammation. In open wounds, exosome secretion of cytokine influences the cellular behavior of fibroblasts toward wound healing.

In pulmonary arterial hypertension (PAH), depletion of pulmonary caveolin-1 from the lungs is partially due to caveolin-1 positive extracellular vesicle (bigger than 100 nm) blebbing and shedding into the circulation [55]. Elevated levels of blood caveolin-1 + EVs correlated with TGF-β-induced microvascular remodeling and PAH [55]. In PAH, the vascular injury most probably induces EV release and caveolin-1 depletion from pulmonary ECs, while the "second hit" that promotes vascular remodeling might be chronic hypoxia [55]. In acute lung injury (ALI), EVs released by vascular ECs and epithelial cells in the lung has been shown to mediate cell-to-cell communication and transport bioactive molecules between cells. However, the role of bioactive proteins and lipid mediators carried by EVs in ALI pathophysiology is explored insufficiently. Mouse bronchoalveolar lavage fluid-derived EVs were found to contain high levels of cyclooxygenase, lipoxygenase, and cytochrome p450 metabolites, those levels increase during the acute inflammatory phase and decrease in the resolution phase of LPS-induced ALI.

Exosomes derived from apoptotic ECs have a particular secretome output, they contain self-made, self-tailored, non-coding RNAs and are ***highly immunogenic***. Apoptotic ECs exosomes are carrying RNAs that are not usually found in healthy cells: viral-like endogenous retroelements (those are the most abundant), mitochondrial

RNAs, U1 small nuclear RNA, and Y RNA that are involved in autoimmunity responses [56]. These nucleic acids are rich in U-bases and unstable folded, self-made RNAs of endothelial cells in apoptosis that can be recognized by toll-like receptors (TLR3, 7, and 8). They encompass a demonstrated role in murine models of inflammation and innate immune responses [56].

MiRNA-enriched EVs derived from monocytes can be transfer to quiescent, unstimulated ECs, which enhanced EC permeability and monocyte transmigration in a co-culture system condition.

In an *in vitro* study, Li et al. employed a co-culture system in which neutrophils extracted from healthy donor blood were co-cultured with brain microvascular ECs in presence of LPS. Exosomes purified from the LPS- exposed miR-122-5p rich neutrophils regulate oxidative stress, permeability, or apoptosis of capillary ECs in the brain [57].

miRNA-containing EVs originating from activated or apoptotic EC are able to communicate to their neighbors, are protecting the adjacent vascular ECs from apoptosis, and have potent ***anti-inflammatory effects*** [58]. Endothelial MVs transporting miR222 to the neighboring ECs are significantly reducing the ICAM-1 level in proximity cells, which have impaired monocyte adhesion assay [59]. *In vitro*, the pretreatment with EC-derived EVs (obtained from ECs stimulated with TNF-α) lead to reduced endothelial ICAM-1 expression at mRNA and protein levels, while did not influence VCAM1 [59]. *In vivo*, they were also able to demonstrate reduced ICAM-1 expression in APO E−/−mice, as shown by immunostaining assays of fragments of descending aorta from APO E−/−mice [59]. These protective effects of EC-derived EVs occurred by delivery of miRNA-222 to recipient endothelial cells [59]. The efficient delivery of miRNA-222 to the recipient cells was demonstrated by employing an assay developed from C. elegans, HCAEC were transfected with cel-miR-39 [59]. Next, they applied prediction methods questioning the target mRNA for miRNA222, and the most probable target was found by ICAM1 [59]. By using inhibitors of miRNA222 they were able to verify that functional miRNA222 targets ICAM1 and reduces its mRNA and protein expression in cultured cells [59, 60].

In an unstimulated, quiescent state, vascular ECs secrete extracellular vesicles containing anti-inflammatory microRNAs [57, 61]. They are transferring miRNA to monocytes and other vascular cells to prevent monocyte activation [62].

EC-derived EVs that can transfer MiR-10a to monocytic/macrophagic cells have anti-inflammatory effects. They inhibit the proinflammatory phenotype by inhibiting many proinflammatory genes by repressing the induction of the nuclear factor-kB (NF-kB) and IRF5 transcriptional pathways. MiR-10a negatively regulates effector proteins that destabilize I-kB. EC-derived EVs that can transfer MiR-10a to monocytic/macrophagic cells suppress a network of genes. One of these genes is interleukin-1-receptor-associated-kinase-4 (IRAK4) gene, which acts upstream of NF-kB signaling. MiR-10a suppressed β-TRC, and MAP3K7/TAK1 [62]. Loss of miR10 during atherogenesis has the opposite effect of activation of monocytes [63].

Increased/disturbed shear flow may lead ECs to deliver miRNAs miR126-3p, miR200a-3p to target cells like smooth muscle cells (SMC) by means *independent of membrane-bound vesicles* and argonaute-2-dependent, which is protecting miRNAs during delivery to the target cells [64] via VAMP-3/SNAP23-mediated pathway, leading to SMC hyperplasia.

Endothelial cell-specific MiR-126 decreased inflammatory-inducible expression of adhesion molecules in ECs, it decreased TNFα-induced VCAM-1 level in cultured primary human ECs, respectively, as shown by immunoblotting [65]. The presence of proinflammatory cytokines, such as TNF-a, induce the expression of VCAM-1 through the induction of NFkB and IRF1 pathway [65]. It has been suggested that miR126 is a target for VCAM-1 gene because of partial sequence matching in the 3' UTR region position 619 to 625 within the human VCAM-1 transcript [65]. Transfection of HUVECs with antisense miR126 increased TNFα-induced VCAM-1 expression [65]. Overexpression of premiR-126, a precursor of miR126 increased endogenous miR126 and reduced VCAM1 expression [65]. Endothelial cell-specific MiR-126 negatively regulates leukocyte trafficking and adherence to TNF-α-activated HUVECs, through VCAM-1 expression inhibition [65]; the leukocyte rolling is VCAM-1 dependent, as shown by blocking VCAM-1 with an anti-VCAM-1 antibody [65, 66].

Primary rat hepatocyte-derived, CD81 and CD63 positive EVs were found to contain argininase-1, an enzyme that regulates the level of arginine, the substrate for eNOS nitric oxide synthetase [67, 68]. *In vivo*, these hepatic EVs obtained from the serum of rats under liver-damaging conditions with acetaminophen, or diclofenac treatment encapsulate more arginase-1 compared to untreated control [67], as shown by the untargeted blood metabolome approach [68]. Exposure of rat pulmonary artery ECs to hepatic EVs for 2 h provoked changes in ECs metabolome as compared to untreated control EVs, via an arginase-1-dependent mechanism [67]. Increased arginase activity led to nitric oxide defective synthesis and activity and ECs malfunction of pulmonary arteries in rats treated with liver-damaging drugs [67].

A screening (Taqman miRNA assay) for high levels of miRNAs in circulating vesicles collected from 180 patients with chronic coronary disease and circa 60 patients with the acute coronary syndrome, identified miRNA-92a-3p to be selectively increased in circulating vesicles isolated from plasma of patients with the coronary disease compared with control, as seen by RT-PCR [69], showing how atherosclerotic conditions selectively promote packaging of miRNAs, such as miRNA-92a-3p into circulating EVs [69]. The authors further explored the role of circulating vesicles carrying miRNAs on vascular ECs [69]. Functional miRNA-92a-3p was transferred from circulating vesicles into acceptor ECs [69]. MiR-92a-3p target is thrombospondin-1, which is increasing cell proliferation and migration, and inhibited angiogenesis and vessel-like networks [69].

Weilner et al. observed a higher rate of exosome secretion in senescent humans ECs compared with quiescent cells [70]. Circulating miR-31, encapsulated by senescent human EC-derived EVs, is upregulated in elderly donors and osteoporosis patients [70]. MiR-31-rich EV transfer in human mesenchymal stem cells inhibiting their differentiation toward osteogenesis, a switch from osteoblast genesis to osteoclast formation, which modifies the bone density [70]. Endothelial exosomes can transfer miR-503 to tumor cells, tumor cells can exert an antitumor effect via the transfer of miRNA from ECs, leading to decreased tumor growth and invasion [70].

4. Role of endothelial Secretome in vascular repair

EVs from ischemic tissues play a role in endothelial cell survival and in *de novo,* angiogenesis as shown in a murine model of ischemia after femoral artery ligation [47, 71]. Hussein et al. showed that injured ECs release caspase 3-rich EVs to protect the endothelial cells from complement-induced apoptosis in cultured HUVECs. Conversely, in the presence of inhibitors like staurosporine they showed that caspase

3 levels increase [71]. Thus, endothelial-derived MV contributes to the elimination of excess, stress levels of apoptotic agents, and to avoid apoptosis and cellular detachment [71].

Endothelial cells react to stressful conditions by releasing EVs, as a form of communicating the distress to the cells in proximity and to protect the endothelium [46]. Under lipid-induced oxidative stress conditions, endothelial cells release EVs containing endothelial NO synthase via AKT/eNOS -dependent signaling pathway, to protect the vessel from endothelial damage [46].

Secretory granules and vesicles can release mediators that are directly involved in the gatekeeper actions of EC by immediate, basal, or by evoked, rapid secretion according to the functional needs of the ECs. CD47 is an integrin-associated protein found often on EVs. CD47 role is to prevent EVs phagocytosis by macrophages, therefore, increasing EVs circulation time [15]. Moreover, activated protein-C (APC) interacts with endothelial protein-C receptor (EPCR) exposed both on the MVs surface and on ECs can cleave PAR-1 and trigger signaling leading to activation of S1P1 which via PI3 and AKT-dependent transactivation of KDR stimulate cell proliferation, and ultimately has an endothelial barrier and cytoprotective effects [72].

Endothelial-derived MV contributes to the sorting of several proapoptotic factors preventing cell detachment and apoptosis [71]. MVs carrying APC induced cytoprotective effects in a staurosporine-induced endothelial cell model of apoptosis assessed by APOPercentage assay and improved EC permeability percentage [72]. Activated protein-C (APC) binding to endothelial protein-C receptor (EPCR) exposed both on the MVs surface and on ECs can cleave PAR-1 and trigger signaling leading to activation of S1P1 which via PI3 and AKT-dependent transactivation of KDR, which, in turn, stimulate cell proliferation, with endothelial barrier protective and EC survival effects [72].

Endothelial exosomes are thought to be involved in angiogenesis. They incorporate and transfer delta-like-4 (Dll4), a notch ligand upregulated during angiogenesis, to neighboring endothelial cells via EVs, beyond cell–cell contact, conferring a tip cell phenotype to the detriment of stalk cells, resulting in a low level of notch signaling, loss of notch receptor and increased filopodia, branching formation that results in neovascularization [73].

Delivery of functional miRNAs by means of ECs-derived EVs to recipient ECs was also shown to help the process of ***vascular repair and angiogenesis*** [74]. In response to hypoxia, the expression of miRNAs, such as miR-210, is upregulated, leading to VEGF-induced chemotaxis to form capillary-like structures in cultured ECs. Upregulation of MiR-210 expression was also found in a surgical murine model of myocardial infarction [75].

5. Discussion and conclusions

By means of their vast secretome, ECs delivery platform sends messages at a distance to circulating blood cells, to other ECs, or to the normal or diseased cells of other organs. ECs complex intercellular communication is possible through the secretory pathways. ECs secretome output may vary, according to the specific vascular bed, whereas ECs phenotype is dictated by their function particularities. The secretome of WPBs is orchestrated by complex, dynamic secretory pathways to meet the versatility of ECs pathophysiology [30]. Novel protein members of the WPBs secretome were recently identified through a new approach of proximity proteomics, unveiling new facets of WPB exocytosis regulation.

EC-derived EVs are primary effectors in signaling pathways between vascular cells. EVs transfer their cargo from the parent cell to the target cell by: (1) docking to the target cell, and (2) internalization of EVs first, before releasing their content. A pool of internalized EVs by the acceptor (target) cells are sent through an endosomal escape system to unusual delivery destinations [13] and (3) release of EV cargo into the cytosol of the acceptor cell, followed by degradation or return to secretion circuit of the vesicles.

The EVs are secreted by virtually all kinds of eukaryotic cells and in all body tissues and fluids, including blood, saliva, urine, amniotic fluid, cerebrospinal fluid, and breast milk. EVs delivery to the target cells may occur using a cell-specific endocytotic mechanism, dependent on receptor-ligand interactions, via clathrin-dependent endocytosis, via clathrin-independent endocytosis lipid rafts-mediated or caveolae-mediated endocytosis, or by common targeting, occurring through pinocytosis, or phagocytosis. It can occur through membrane fusion or via intraluminal vesicles fusion with the endosomal limiting membrane. The sort of the uptake mechanism is given in part by the types of molecular regulators found both on EVs and the targeted plasma membrane of the acceptor cells, because this molecular pair influences the phenotypic traits and behavior of the recipient cells post EV content uptake. Upon shear stress, pH, pressure change, or shock, the ECs release a system of vesicles either into the extracellular space or they reach an additional target cell, which is transformed by this interaction, and that target cell takes on the characteristics of the shredded parent cell.

The ectodomain shedding by proteolytic cleavage of transmembranar protein exterior domain is the posttranslational modification that permits the appearance of new fragments, that function either as receptors or ligands, that control levels of signaling proteins in the recipient cells. This process is not an exemption for transmembranar protein, it rather occurs frequently and is a form of communication between cells. There are still many things unclear about the processes of ectodomain shedding, one question that remains to be elucidated is how the molecular pairing occurs between sheddases and substrates, timing, kinetics, and how sheddases alter the substrate's function and we still must explore their potential as drug targets.

Further, we discussed some aspects related to the posttranscriptional-mediated miRNA regulation of gene expression programs of endothelial cells and their impact on vascular disease. Under disturbed shear flow, miRNAs may be delivered dependent on membrane-bound microparticles [66], or independent of membrane-bound microparticles, with the help of argonaute-2, which protects the miRNAs during delivery to the recipient cells [76].

EVs have beneficial effects, such as anti-inflammatory effects, inhibition of thrombus formation, or vascular repair and angiogenesis [77], but they might have detrimental effects leading to systemic inflammation, atherosclerosis, tilting vascular homeostasis, and thrombotic propensity. Therefore, they could serve as biomarkers of endothelial dysfunction.

EC-derived EVs are frequently found in patients with vascular conditions. EVs found in the plasma of these patients could be used as prognostic factors of vascular disease. Exosomes are still used only in investigational protocols. There are several clinical trials going on trying to prove applications in dermatology (burns) through regeneration and wound healing mediated by exosomes. Some tissular cells can be distinguished from the bloodstream circulating exosomes, but further investigations are needed to delineate the origin of the exosomes in circulation as well as different many facets involved in the creation of the exosomes, in the targeting, transport, and uptake mechanisms (ubiquitin and lipid-mediated) in physiological vs. specific cardiovascular disease condition.

The key advances of endothelial EVs and in particular exosomes for therapeutic purposes are: 1) exosomes can home, 2) can travel systemically without risk of clumping, 3) can travel via local or topical therapy, 4) exosomes cross the "blood–brain barrier," 5) not perceived as foreign, and 6) they deliver miRNA and mRNA and signaling proteins to unite, to mobilize, to integrate, and cytoskeletal proteins to direct the focal adhesion, for matrix-directed acquisition, reduction of proliferation, and matrix production in the target tissue, and cell motion, cell-cycle, anti-apoptotic, and responses to oxidative stress are only a few of the things exosomes can do. 7) No first-pass lung effect, 8) easy to administer, store, and freeze, and 9) the dosage can be controlled.

Further investigations are required to subcategorize the exosomes depending on the cell type or lineage that they are secreted from, and their specific impact on the functions of the vasculature.

A dynamic endothelial cell secretome meets the vasculature bed functional needs through complex secretory pathways EC secretome's constituents could be a readily accessible, rich source of non-toxic markers to monitor and properly assess the risk factors of vascular disease and prognosis. Most importantly, ECs secretome therapeutic potential is emerging for the treatment of various diseases and tissue injuries.

Author details

Luiza Rusu
University of Illinois at Chicago, Chicago, Illinois, USA

*Address all correspondence to: lsergh2@uic.edu

References

[1] Aird WC. Endothelium as an organ system. Critical Care Medicine. 2004;**32**(Suppl. 5):S271-S279

[2] Dragt BS, van Agtmaal EL, de Laat B, Voorberg J. Effect of laminar shear stress on the distribution of Weibel-Palade bodies in endothelial cells. Thrombosis Research. 2012;**130**(5):741-745

[3] Tunica DG, Yin X, Sidibe A, Stegemann C, Nissum M, Zeng L, et al. Proteomic analysis of the secretome of human umbilical vein endothelial cells using a combination of free-flow electrophoresis and nanoflow LC-MS/MS. Proteomics. 2009;**9**(21):4991-4996

[4] Charreau B. Secretome and Tunneling nanotubes: A multilevel network for long range intercellular communication between endothelial cells and distant cells. International Journal of Molecular Sciences. 2021;**22**(15):7971-7994

[5] Holthenrich A, Drexler HCA, Chehab T, Naß J, Gerke V. Proximity proteomics of endothelial Weibel-Palade bodies identifies novel regulator of von Willebrand factor secretion. Blood. 2019;**134**(12):979-982

[6] Hayashida K, Bartlett AH, Chen Y, Park PW. Molecular and cellular mechanisms of ectodomain shedding. The Anatomical Record. 2010;**293**(6):925-937

[7] van Breevoort D, van Agtmaal EL, Dragt BS, Gebbinck JK, Dienava-Verdoold I, Kragt A, et al. Proteomic screen identifies IGFBP7 as a novel component of endothelial cell-specific Weibel-Palade bodies. Journal of Proteome Research. 2012;**11**(5):2925-2936

[8] Ruggeri ZM. Von Willebrand factor, platelets and endothelial cell interactions. Journal of Thrombosis and Haemostasis. 2003;**1**(7):1335-1342

[9] György B, Módos K, Pállinger E, Pálóczi K, Pásztói M, Misják P, et al. Detection and isolation of cell-derived microparticles are compromised by protein complexes resulting from shared biophysical parameters. Blood. 2011;**117**(4):e39-e48

[10] Tkach M, Théry C. Communication by extracellular vesicles: Where we are and where we need to go. Cell. 2016;**164**(6):1226-1232

[11] Kowal J, Tkach M, Théry C. Biogenesis and secretion of exosomes. Current Opinion in Cell Biology. 2014;**29**:116-125

[12] Théry C, Witwer KW, Aikawa E, Alcaraz MJ, Anderson JD, Andriantsitohaina R, et al. Minimal information for studies of extracellular vesicles 2018 (MISEV2018): A position statement of the International Society for Extracellular Vesicles and update of the MISEV2014 guidelines. Journal of Extracellular Vesicles. 2018;**7**(1):1535750

[13] Mathieu M, Martin-Jaular L, Lavieu G, Théry C. Specificities of secretion and uptake of exosomes and other extracellular vesicles for cell-to-cell communication. Nature Cell Biology. 2019;**21**(1):9-17

[14] Mathieu M, Névo N, Jouve M, Valenzuela JI, Maurin M, Verweij FJ, et al. Specificities of exosome versus small ectosome secretion revealed by live intracellular tracking of CD63 and CD9. Nature Communications. 2021;**12**(1):4389

[15] Colombo M, Raposo G, Théry C. Biogenesis, secretion, and intercellular

interactions of exosomes and other extracellular vesicles. Annual Review of Cell and Developmental Biology. 2014;**30**:255-289

[16] Muralidharan-Chari V, Clancy J, Plou C, Romao M, Chavrier P, Raposo G, et al. ARF6-regulated shedding of tumor cell-derived plasma membrane microvesicles. Current Biology. 2009;**19**(22):1875-1885

[17] Weibel ER, Palade GE. New cytoplasmic components in arterial endothelia. The Journal of Cell Biology. 1964;**23**:101-112

[18] Denis C, Methia N, Frenette PS, Rayburn H, Ullman-Cullere M, Hynes RO, et al. A mouse model of severe von Willebrand disease: Defects in hemostasis and thrombosis. Proceedings of the National Academy of Sciences of the United States of America. 1998;**95**(16):9524-9529

[19] Voorberg J, Fontijn R, Calafat J, Janssen H, van Mourik JA, Pannekoek H. Biogenesis of von Willebrand factor-containing organelles in heterologous transfected CV-1 cells. The EMBO Journal. 1993;**12**(2):749-758

[20] Wagner DD, Saffaripour S, Bonfanti R, Sadler JE, Cramer EM, Chapman B, et al. Induction of specific storage organelles by von Willebrand factor propolypeptide. Cell. 1991;**64**(2):403-413

[21] Valentijn KM, Eikenboom J. Weibel-Palade bodies: A window to von Willebrand disease. Journal of Thrombosis and Haemostasis. 2013;**11**(4):581-592

[22] Wagner DD, Marder VJ. Biosynthesis of von Willebrand protein by human endothelial cells: Processing steps and their intracellular localization. The Journal of Cell Biology. 1984;**99**(6): 2123-2130

[23] Vischer UM, Wagner DD. von Willebrand factor proteolytic processing and multimerization precede the formation of Weibel-Palade bodies. Blood. 1994;**83**(12):3536-3544

[24] Sporn LA, Marder VJ, Wagner DD. Inducible secretion of large, biologically potent von Willebrand factor multimers. Cell. 1986;**46**(2):185-190

[25] Zenner HL, Collinson LM, Michaux G, Cutler DF. High-pressure freezing provides insights into Weibel-Palade body biogenesis. Journal of Cell Science. 2007;**120**(Pt 12):2117-2125

[26] Lui-Roberts WW, Collinson LM, Hewlett LJ, Michaux G, Cutler DF. An AP-1/clathrin coat plays a novel and essential role in forming the Weibel-Palade bodies of endothelial cells. The Journal of Cell Biology. 2005;**170**(4):627-636

[27] Vischer UM, Wagner DD. CD63 is a component of Weibel-Palade bodies of human endothelial cells. Blood. 1993;**82**(4):1184-1191

[28] Giblin JP, Hewlett LJ, Hannah MJ. Basal secretion of von Willebrand factor from human endothelial cells. Blood. 2008;**112**(4):957-964

[29] Matsushita K, Morrell CN, Cambien B, Yang SX, Yamakuchi M, Bao C, et al. Nitric oxide regulates exocytosis by S-nitrosylation of N-ethylmaleimide-sensitive factor. Cell. 2003;**115**(2):139-150

[30] Rondaij MG, Bierings R, Kragt A, van Mourik JA, Voorberg J. Dynamics and plasticity of Weibel-Palade bodies in endothelial cells. Arteriosclerosis, Thrombosis, and Vascular Biology. 2006;**26**(5):1002-1007

[31] Bonfanti R, Furie BC, Furie B, Wagner DD. PADGEM (GMP140) is a component of Weibel-Palade bodies of human endothelial cells. Blood. 1989;**73**(5):1109-1112

[32] Padilla A, Moake JL, Bernardo A, Ball C, Wang Y, Arya M, et al. P-selectin anchors newly released ultralarge von Willebrand factor multimers to the endothelial cell surface. Blood. 2004;**103**(6):2150-2156

[33] Denis CV, André P, Saffaripour S, Wagner DD. Defect in regulated secretion of P-selectin affects leukocyte recruitment in von Willebrand factor-deficient mice. Proceedings of the National Academy of Sciences of the United States of America. 2001;**98**(7):4072-4077

[34] Pendu R, Terraube V, Christophe OD, Gahmberg CG, de Groot PG, Lenting PJ, et al. P-selectin glycoprotein ligand 1 and beta2-integrins cooperate in the adhesion of leukocytes to von Willebrand factor. Blood. 2006;**108**(12):3746-3752

[35] Rosenberg JB, Greengard JS, Montgomery RR. Genetic induction of a releasable pool of factor VIII in human endothelial cells. Arteriosclerosis, Thrombosis, and Vascular Biology. 2000;**20**(12):2689-2695

[36] Simonet WS, Lacey DL, Dunstan CR, Kelley M, Chang MS, Lüthy R, et al. Osteoprotegerin: A novel secreted protein involved in the regulation of bone density. Cell. 1997;**89**(2):309-319

[37] Starke RD, Ferraro F, Paschalaki KE, Dryden NH, McKinnon TA, Sutton RE, et al. Endothelial von Willebrand factor regulates angiogenesis. Blood. 2011;**117**(3):1071-1080

[38] Bierings R, Hellen N, Kiskin N, Knipe L, Fonseca AV, Patel B, et al. The interplay between the Rab27A effectors Slp4-a and MyRIP controls hormone-evoked Weibel-Palade body exocytosis. Blood. 2012;**120**(13):2757-2767

[39] Zhou HJ, Qin L, Zhang H, Tang W, Ji W, He Y, et al. Erratum: Endothelial exocytosis of angiopoietin-2 resulting from CCM3 deficiency contributes to cerebral cavernous malformation. Nature Medicine. 2016;**22**(12):1502

[40] Knipe L, Meli A, Hewlett L, Bierings R, Dempster J, Skehel P, et al. A revised model for the secretion of tPA and cytokines from cultured endothelial cells. Blood. 2010;**116**(12):2183-2191

[41] Hol J, Küchler AM, Johansen FE, Dalhus B, Haraldsen G, Oynebråten I. Molecular requirements for sorting of the chemokine interleukin-8/CXCL8 to endothelial Weibel-Palade bodies. The Journal of Biological Chemistry. 2009;**284**(35):23532-23539

[42] Øynebråten I, Bakke O, Brandtzaeg P, Johansen FE, Haraldsen G. Rapid chemokine secretion from endothelial cells originates from 2 distinct compartments. Blood. 2004;**104**(2):314-320

[43] Øynebråten I, Barois N, Hagelsteen K, Johansen FE, Bakke O, Haraldsen G. Characterization of a novel chemokine-containing storage granule in endothelial cells: Evidence for preferential exocytosis mediated by protein kinase a and diacylglycerol. Journal of Immunology. 2005;**175**(8):5358-5369

[44] Chatterjee V, Yang X, Ma Y, Cha B, Meegan JE, Wu M, et al. Endothelial microvesicles carrying Src-rich cargo impair adherens junction integrity and cytoskeleton homeostasis. Cardiovascular Research. 2020;**116**(8):1525-1538

[45] Chironi GN, Boulanger CM, Simon A, Dignat-George F, Freyssinet JM, Tedgui A. Endothelial microparticles in diseases. Cell and Tissue Research. 2009;**335**(1):143-151

[46] Mathiesen A, Hamilton T, Carter N, Brown M, McPheat W, Dobrian A. Endothelial extracellular vesicles: From keepers of health to messengers of disease. International Journal of Molecular Sciences. 2021;**22**(9):4640-4666

[47] Leroyer AS, Ebrahimian TG, Cochain C, Récalde A, Blanc-Brude O, Mees B, et al. Microparticles from ischemic muscle promotes postnatal vasculogenesis. Circulation. 2009;**119**(21):2808-2817

[48] Colombo M, Moita C, van Niel G, Kowal J, Vigneron J, Benaroch P, et al. Analysis of ESCRT functions in exosome biogenesis, composition and secretion highlights the heterogeneity of extracellular vesicles. Journal of Cell Science. 2013;**126**(Pt 24):5553-5565

[49] Jaé N, McEwan DG, Manavski Y, Boon RA, Dimmeler S. Rab7a and Rab27b control secretion of endothelial microRNA through extracellular vesicles. FEBS Letters. 2015;**589**(20 Pt B): 3182-3188

[50] Hundhausen C, Schulte A, Schulz B, Andrzejewski MG, Schwarz N, von Hundelshausen P, et al. Regulated shedding of transmembrane chemokines by the disintegrin and metalloproteinase 10 facilitates detachment of adherent leukocytes. Journal of Immunology. 2007;**178**(12):8064-8072

[51] Pabois A, Devallière J, Quillard T, Coulon F, Gérard N, Laboisse C, et al. The disintegrin and metalloproteinase ADAM10 mediates a canonical notch-dependent regulation of IL-6 through Dll4 in human endothelial cells. Biochemical Pharmacology. 2014;**91**(4):510-521

[52] Schulz B, Pruessmeyer J, Maretzky T, Ludwig A, Blobel CP, Saftig P, et al. ADAM10 regulates endothelial permeability and T-cell transmigration by proteolysis of vascular endothelial cadherin. Circulation Research. 2008;**102**(10):1192-1201

[53] Yang J, LeBlanc ME, Cano I, Saez-Torres KL, Saint-Geniez M, Ng YS, et al. ADAM10 and ADAM17 proteases mediate proinflammatory cytokine-induced and constitutive cleavage of endomucin from the endothelial surface. The Journal of Biological Chemistry. 2020;**295**(19):6641-6651

[54] Pabois A, Pagie S, Gérard N, Laboisse C, Pattier S, Hulin P, et al. Notch signaling mediates crosstalk between endothelial cells and macrophages via Dll4 and IL6 in cardiac microvascular inflammation. Biochemical Pharmacology. 2016;**104**:95-107

[55] Oliveira SDS, Chen J, Castellon M, Mao M, Raj JU, Comhair S, et al. Injury-induced shedding of extracellular vesicles depletes endothelial cells of Cav-1 (Caveolin-1) and enables TGF-β (transforming growth factor-β)-dependent pulmonary arterial hypertension. Arteriosclerosis, Thrombosis, and Vascular Biology. 2019;**39**(6):1191-1202

[56] Hardy MP, Audemard É, Migneault F, Feghaly A, Brochu S, Gendron P, et al. Apoptotic endothelial cells release small extracellular vesicles loaded with immunostimulatory viral-like RNAs. Scientific Reports. 2019;**9**(1):7203

[57] Li Q, Nong A, Huang Z, Xu Y, He K, Jia Y, et al. Exosomes containing miR-122-5p secreted by LPS-induced neutrophils regulate the apoptosis and

permeability of brain microvascular endothelial cells by targeting OCLN. American Journal of Translational Research. 2021;**13**(5):4167-4181

[58] Jansen F, Yang X, Proebsting S, Hoelscher M, Przybilla D, Baumann K, et al. MicroRNA expression in circulating microvesicles predicts cardiovascular events in patients with coronary artery disease. Journal of the American Heart Association. 2014;**3**(6):e001249

[59] Jansen F, Yang X, Baumann K, Przybilla D, Schmitz T, Flender A, et al. Endothelial microparticles reduce ICAM-1 expression in a microRNA-222-dependent mechanism. Journal of Cellular and Molecular Medicine. 2015;**19**(9):2202-2214

[60] Jansen F, Zietzer A, Stumpf T, Flender A, Schmitz T, Nickenig G, et al. Endothelial microparticle-promoted inhibition of vascular remodeling is abrogated under hyperglycaemic conditions. Journal of Molecular and Cellular Cardiology. 2017;**112**:91-94

[61] Nong A, Li Q, Huang Z, Xu Y, He K, Jia Y, et al. MicroRNA miR-126 attenuates brain injury in septic rats via NF-κB signaling pathway. Bioengineered. 2021;**12**(1):2639-2648

[62] Njock MS, Cheng HS, Dang LT, Nazari-Jahantigh M, Lau AC, Boudreau E, et al. Endothelial cells suppress monocyte activation through secretion of extracellular vesicles containing antiinflammatory microRNAs. Blood. 2015;**125**(20):3202-3212

[63] Fang Y, Shi C, Manduchi E, Civelek M, Davies PF. MicroRNA-10a regulation of proinflammatory phenotype in athero-susceptible endothelium in vivo and in vitro. Proceedings of the National Academy of Sciences of the United States of America. 2010;**107**(30):13450-13455

[64] Zhou J, Li YS, Nguyen P, Wang KC, Weiss A, Kuo YC, et al. Regulation of vascular smooth muscle cell turnover by endothelial cell-secreted microRNA-126: Role of shear stress. Circulation Research. 2013;**113**(1):40-51

[65] Harris TA, Yamakuchi M, Ferlito M, Mendell JT, Lowenstein CJ. MicroRNA-126 regulates endothelial expression of vascular cell adhesion molecule 1. Proceedings of the National Academy of Sciences of the United States of America. 2008;**105**(5):1516-1521

[66] Fernández-Hernando C, Suárez Y. MicroRNAs in endothelial cell homeostasis and vascular disease. Current Opinion in Hematology. 2018;**25**(3):227-236

[67] Royo F, Moreno L, Mleczko J, Palomo L, Gonzalez E, Cabrera D, et al. Hepatocyte-secreted extracellular vesicles modify blood metabolome and endothelial function by an arginase-dependent mechanism. Scientific Reports. 2017;**7**:42798

[68] Palomo L, Casal E, Royo F, Cabrera D, van-Liempd S, Falcon-Perez JM. Considerations for applying metabolomics to the analysis of extracellular vesicles. Frontiers in Immunology. 2014;**5**:651

[69] Liu Y, Li Q, Hosen MR, Zietzer A, Flender A, Levermann P, et al. Atherosclerotic conditions promote the packaging of functional MicroRNA-92a-3p into endothelial microvesicles. Circulation Research. 2019;**124**(4):575-587

[70] Weilner S, Schraml E, Wieser M, Messner P, Schneider K, Wassermann K,

et al. Secreted microvesicular miR-31 inhibits osteogenic differentiation of mesenchymal stem cells. Aging Cell. 2016;**15**(4):744-754

[71] Abid Hussein MN, Böing AN, Sturk A, Hau CM, Nieuwland R. Inhibition of microparticle release triggers endothelial cell apoptosis and detachment. Thrombosis and Haemostasis. 2007;**98**(5):1096-1107

[72] Pérez-Casal M, Downey C, Cutillas-Moreno B, Zuzel M, Fukudome K, Toh CH. Microparticle-associated endothelial protein C receptor and the induction of cytoprotective and anti-inflammatory effects. Haematologica. 2009;**94**(3):387-394

[73] Sheldon H, Heikamp E, Turley H, Dragovic R, Thomas P, Oon CE, et al. New mechanism for notch signaling to endothelium at a distance by Delta-like 4 incorporation into exosomes. Blood. 2010;**116**(13):2385-2394

[74] Jansen F, Stumpf T, Proebsting S, Franklin BS, Wenzel D, Pfeifer P, et al. Intercellular transfer of miR-126-3p by endothelial microparticles reduces vascular smooth muscle cell proliferation and limits neointima formation by inhibiting LRP6. Journal of Molecular and Cellular Cardiology. 2017;**104**: 43-52

[75] Hu S, Huang M, Li Z, Jia F, Ghosh Z, Lijkwan MA, et al. MicroRNA-210 as a novel therapy for treatment of ischemic heart disease. Circulation. 2010;**122** (11 Suppl):S124-S131

[76] Zhu JJ, Liu YF, Zhang YP, Zhao CR, Yao WJ, Li YS, et al. VAMP3 and SNAP23 mediate the disturbed flow-induced endothelial microRNA secretion and smooth muscle hyperplasia. Proceedings of the National Academy of Sciences of the United States of America. 2017;**114**(31):8271-8276

[77] Cocozza F, Grisard E, Martin-Jaular L, Mathieu M, Théry C. SnapShot: Extracellular vesicles. Cell. 2020;**182**(1):262.e1

Chapter 3

An Insight into Classification, Diagnosis and Comprehensive Management of Food Impaction

Renganath Murugan Jeyasree and Thamilselvan Muthuraj

Abstract

Food impaction is a commonly occurring entity evidenced in day-to-day dental practice. Various factors, such as improperly built proximal restoration, improperly fabricated crown with interdental spacing, opposing plunger cusps, ill-fitting prosthesis and proximal space created after orthodontic treatment by placement of molar bands, act as a reason for food getting impacted in the proximal space of the dentition. But at the same time, it is neglected without knowing the course of pathogenesis of the same, which could eventually lead to formation of localized periodontitis and further progression even leads to loss of dentition. Hence, this chapter gives an in-depth insight to aetiology, clinical and radiographic diagnosis and various means of management of food impaction from a periodontist perspective.

Keywords: food impaction, food lodgement, periodontitis, proximal contact, bone loss

1. Introduction

Food impaction around natural or artificial teeth has become a commonly occurring problem in dentistry. Food impaction occurs when food was forcefully wedged into the periodontium. It is defined as 'the forceful wedging of food into the interproximal space by masticatory pressure (vertical impaction) or the forcing of food interproximally by tongue or cheek pressure (horizontal impaction) defined by glossary of periodontal terms' [1].

Food impaction may be due to anatomical causes or iatrogenic. There was a direct relationship between the contact, contour and shape of the teeth that creates the interproximal space to access path for food to get impacted in between the interproximal spaces.

Food impaction may be vertical or horizontal. Most vertical food impaction is anatomic or clinician induced during fabrication of restoration, whereas horizontal food impaction may be secondary to periodontal disease. It is vertical impaction in which improper pre-operative care, overlooking of certain details and lack of specific knowledge that attributed the problem. Though not entirely surmountable, this chapter gives an insight into sequel of events occurring because of food impaction and may help in mitigating this problem to a small extent.

2. Classification

Hirschfeld [2] has documented several conditions and factors responsible for food impaction and gave a classification of factors causing food impaction, which are as follows:

2.1 Classification of factors causing food impaction (Dr khairnar revised classification of Food impaction)

Class I: Occlusal wear
Class II: Loss of proximal contact
Class III: Extrusion beyond the occlusal plane
Class IV: Congenital morphological abnormality
Class V: Improperly constructed restorations

2.1.1 Class I: occlusal wear

2.1.1.1 Type A

Wedging action is produced by the transformation of occlusal convexities into oblique facets, exaggerating the action of plunger cusp (**Figure 1**) [3].

2.1.1.2 Type B

The distal portion of the maxillary molars exhibits obliquely worn-off structure, which overhangs the distal surface of its functional antagonist. When the cusp of

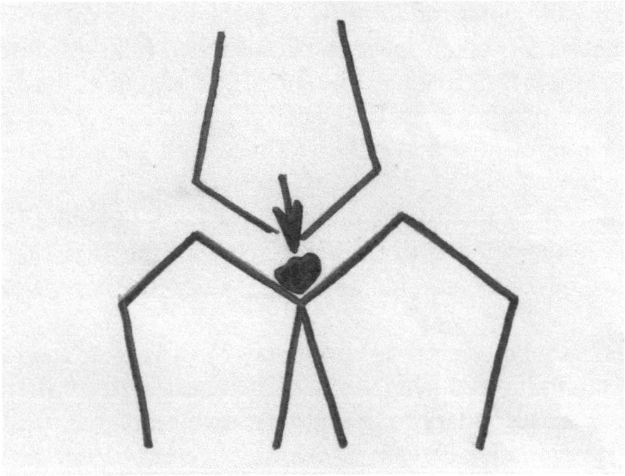

Figure 1.
Wedging action of food by plunger cusp.

maxillary tooth is overhanging the distal surface of mandibular tooth, in such case, the maxillary tooth is forced distally by occlusal forces and bolus of the food, destroying the mesial proximal contact and favours food impaction (**Figure 2**).

2.1.1.3 Type C

Mandibular molars overlap the distal surface of functional antagonist due to obliquely worn tooth structure. When there is attrition on the mesial portion of the crown of the mandibular molar and it is overlapping the distal surface of maxillary molar, due to functional relationship, mandibular molar is forced distally, thus creating open contact at mesial aspect that favours food impaction mesial to mandibular molar (**Figure 3**).

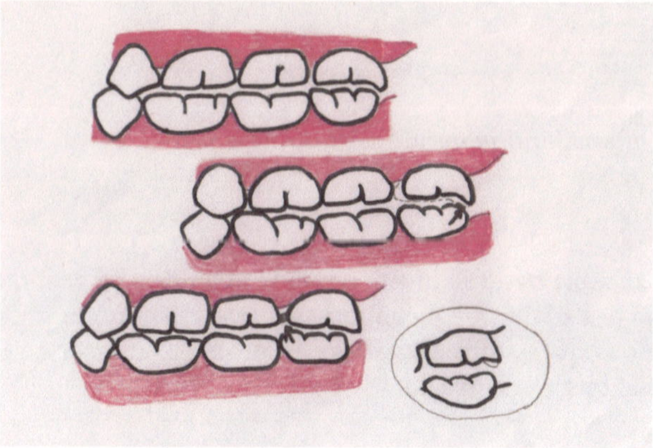

Figure 2.
Maxillary overhanging cusp forcing food in mandibular proximal contact.

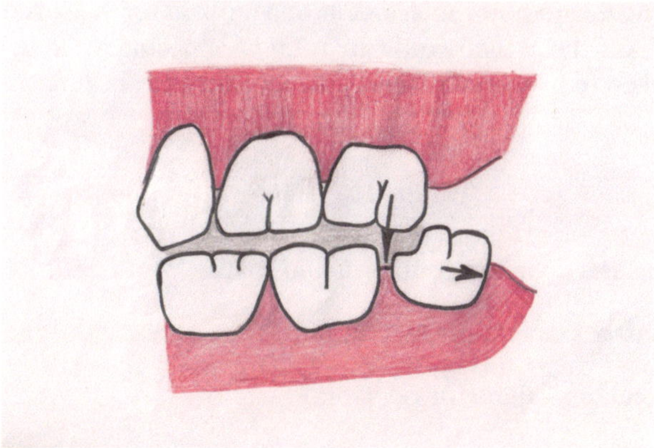

Figure 3.
Obliquely worn mandibular mesial portion favouring food impaction.

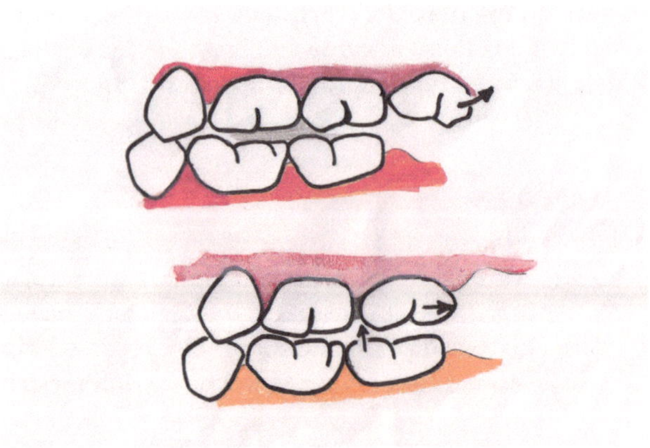

Figure 4.
Open proximal contact mesial to distal tooth and distal to mesial tooth.

2.1.2 Class II: loss of proximal support

2.1.2.1 Type A

Loss of distal support because of the removal of a distal adjacent tooth. Extraction of molar results in loss of proximal support that leads to gradual shifting of adjacent teeth into edentulous space, thus creating open proximal contact mesial to distal tooth and distal to mesial tooth (**Figure 4**).

2.1.2.2 Type B

Loss of mesial support due to the extraction of mesial tooth.

2.1.2.3 Type C

Oblique drifting due to non-replacement of a missing tooth leads to loss of space by drifting of mesial and distal tooth and extrusion of opposing tooth into the edentulous space. This opens up to proximal contact relationship and favours food impaction (**Figure 5**).

2.1.2.4 Type D

Permanent occlusal openings to interdental spaces (**Figure 6**).

i. Drifting after extraction.

ii. Habits forcing teeth out of position.

iii. Periodontal disease.

iv. Caries.

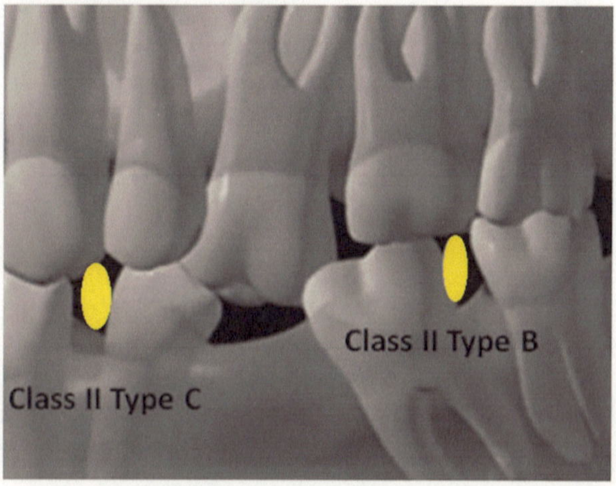

Figure 5.
Teeth drifting due to non-replaced missing tooth.

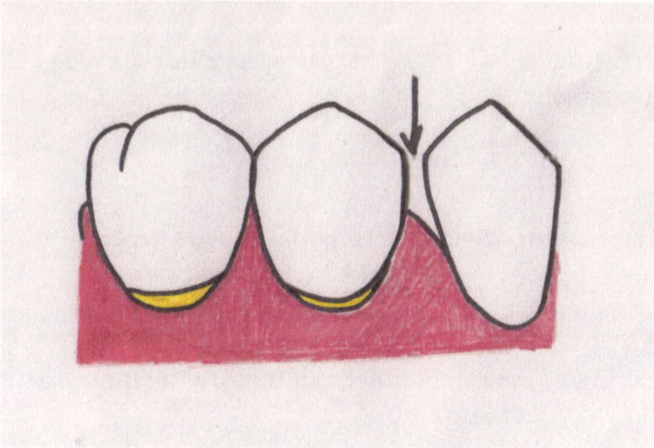

Figure 6.
Permanent occlusal openings to interdental spaces.

2.1.3 Class III: extrusion beyond the occlusal plane

Extrusion of a tooth, which was previously retaining contiguity with the adjacent mesial and distal teeth, results in occlusal step deformity between marginal ridges of extruded and non-extruded teeth. Thus, disturbing proximal contact relationship and favouring food impaction (**Figure** 7).

2.1.4 Class IV: congenital morphologic abnormalities

Any congenital morphologic abnormalities in size, shape, form and position of the tooth leading to open proximal contact were conducive to food impaction.

2.1.4.1 Type A

Position of rotated tooth. Position of tooth with buccal rotation, most commonly premolars with buccal surface facing mesial and lingual surface distally. In such

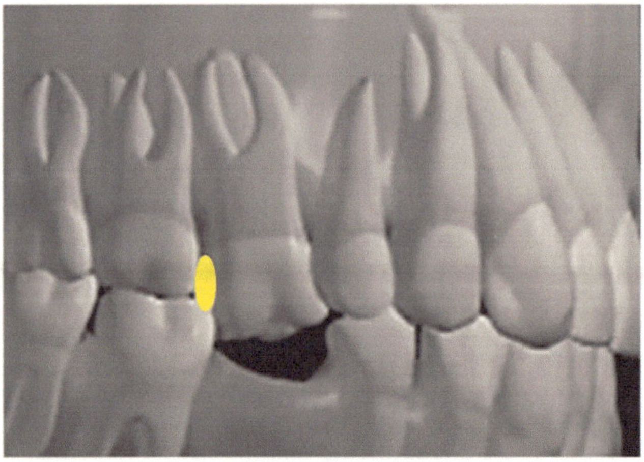

Figure 7.
Extrusion beyond the occlusal plane.

situations, where occlusal surface of premolar was inclined, food gets directed into the distal interproximal space.

2.1.4.2 Type B

Emphasized embrasure between teeth with bulbous neck.

2.1.4.3 Type C

Facio-lingual tilting of the tooth either can modify the interproximal contact with adjacent teeth, allowing food impaction.

2.1.4.4 Type D

Lingual or buccal position of the tooth. Malpositioning of the tooth either more buccally or lingually, especially anterior with a crossbite, can also cause food impaction.

2.1.5 Class V: improperly constructed restoration

2.1.5.1 Type A

Loss of contact point in any restoration or prosthesis permits passage of food into interproximal areas forced by plunger cusp causing further periodontal destruction.

2.1.5.2 Type B

Improper location of contact point. Establishing contact too occlusally will create a smaller occlusal embrasure space. This will prevent food from escaping interproximal region and action of plunger cusp will force the food into interproximal periodontium. Establishment of a contact point too gingivally will induce an inflammatory response in interdental papilla region leading to bone loss.

2.1.5.3 Type C

Improper occlusal contour due to faulty restoration design with establishment of improper flat interproximal contour leads to inappropriate proximal contact and later will progress into food lodgement.

2.1.5.4 Type D

Improperly constructed cantilever restorations.

2.1.5.5 Type E

Tissue-borne areas of prosthetic restorations giving scalloped cervical bevels, that is, the finishing line of the restorations are over contoured at mesial and distal aspects, it may induce periodontitis, leading to loss of interdental bone [3]. Scalloped cervical bevels on finishing margins of prosthetic crowns can be evaluated by running an explorer along the margins of the crown.

3. Occurrence

Jung et al. [4] in a clinical study on the occurrence of food impaction evaluated the following results:

- Teeth without distal support were found to be the most frequent site of food impaction (41.6%).
- Food impaction was found to be more frequent in the upper teeth (66.2%) than in the lower teeth (33.8%).
- Food impaction was found in tight contact cases (71.4%). Alveolar bone loss was not found in the early stage of food impaction (83.1%).
- The distance between the marginal ridges of food impaction sites (mean=0.48 mm) was shorter than that of the control group.
- In 18.2% of the cases, proximal caries were found at the food impaction site.
- Food impaction affected patient's occlusion with the following frequencies: cusp to marginal ridge relationship (72.7%), cusp to fossa relationship (3.9%) and stepped relationship (23.4%).

4. Factors that contribute to food impaction

1. Prosthodontics-periodontal insight
    - Poorly fabricated crown
    - Poorly fabricated partial dentures
    - Improperly constructed implant crowns
2. Conservative dentistry-periodontal insight
    - Unpolished restorations
    - Broken class II restorations
    - Loss of proximal contact restorations
3. Orthodontics-periodontal insight
    - Post-orthodontic treatment induced periodontitis
    - Malocclusion as a factor for food impaction

4.1 Poorly fabricated crown

When the margin of restoration was not properly blended with tooth surface, it gives a space for bacterial accumulation. The proximal finish line preparation should also move along the contour of interdental papilla. But it was commonly prepared as a straight line or a flat margin, thus invading the papillary space, which leads to irritation of the interdental papilla and later may undergo atrophy. In both conditions, it gives rise to food impaction. The under surface of pontic should have passive contact with mucosa. If not, then oral hygiene measures are hindered, causing plaque accumulation and development of periodontal pocket in adjacent tooth, which further leads to horizontal food impaction in that area [5].

4.2 Poorly fabricated partial dentures

Patients wearing removable partial dentures had minor difficulties with the problem of food accumulation in between the partial denture and teeth, most commonly in mandibular removable partial dentures. It was also noted that patients wearing older dentures were more prone to get food accumulation between the denture and teeth interface when compared with patients wearing newer removable partial dentures. It was central to find that removable partial denture wearers got greater degree of plaque index, gingival index and probing depth [6].

4.3 Improperly constructed implant crowns

Proximal contact loss between implant-supported fixed dental prostheses (FDPs) and adjacent teeth has been suggested as a predisposing factor causing food impaction, which in turn leads to an adverse effect on peri-implant tissues [7–9]. Food impaction between implant-supported fixed dental prosthesis and adjacent teeth occurred more frequently when proximal contact was lost and the embrasure surface area (ESA) was greater. Dimensions of the embrasure also influenced the peri-implant mucosal conditions and bone level around the implant [10].

4.4 Unpolished restorations

Rough surfaces of unpolished restoration act as scaffold for plaque accumulation, which later colonizes and becomes a mineralised form of calculus. This, in turn, deepens the gingival sulcus, thus creating inter proximal pocket and attachment, which leads to creation of space for food impaction.

4.5 Broken Class II restorations

It was noted that the problem regarding posterior resin composite restorations was the difficulty in achieving ideal proximal contours and contacts in Class II cavities. Open contacts lead to food impaction and then periodontal disease [11–13].

4.6 Loss of proximal contact

Studies compared periodontal status adjacent to unilateral open contacts and contralateral closed contacts in which food impaction and occlusal interference were significantly more prevalent at open contacts. In addition, 60.6% of patients had greater clinical attachment loss (CAL) and 49% had deeper probing depths (PD) at open contact sites compared to 17.3% CAL and 22.1% deeper PD at closed contact sites [8].

4.7 Post-orthodontic treatment-induced periodontitis

Studies have shown that in the early stages of fixed orthodontic treatment, molar bands are associated with greater periodontal inflammation, exhibiting more bleeding on probing and an increase in periodontal pocket depth when compared with molar bonds [14].

4.8 Malocclusion as a factor for food impaction

Mal-aligned teeth and malocclusion contribute to formation of periodontal disease, especially gingivitis in the initial stages and later into periodontitis. This is because of the fact that mal-aligned teeth and malocclusion consent the accumulation of plaque and calculus around the teeth and this, in turn, leads to well-established gingivitis and further progression into periodontitis with loss of attachment and accumulation of food in the lost periodontal tissue areas [15].

5. Clinical sequelae of food impaction

5.1 Vertical food impaction

Vertical food impaction

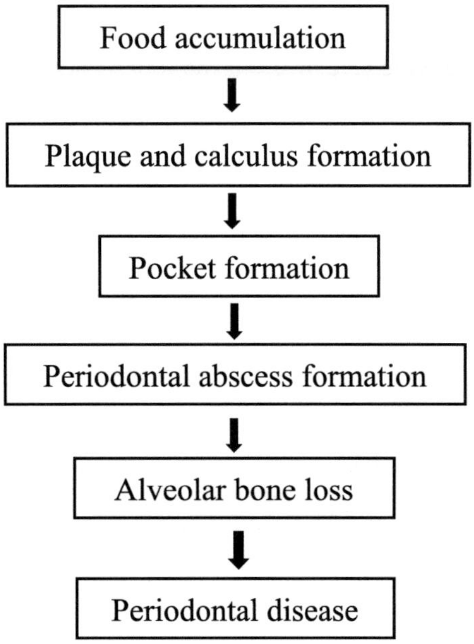

5.2 Horizontal food impaction

Horizontal food impaction

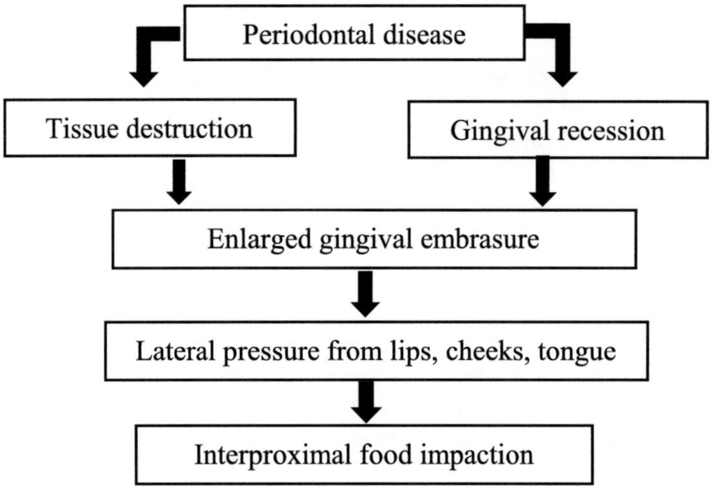

6. Diagnostic methods

6.1 Clinical diagnosis

6.1.1 Detailed history from the patient

It is always essential to take a detailed history from the patient regarding the symptoms the patient encountered from the existing problem. The commonly quoted questions could be as follows:

- *Whether food gets stuck between teeth or gums?*
- *When was the first time the food got stuck?*
- *How long the food lodgement was occurring?*
- *What were the symptoms when food was stuck?*
- *What were the means used to retrieve or remove the trapped food?*
- *Whether any treatment has been undergone before for the same?*

Once the above questions are inquired to the patient, the next and vital step in diagnosis includes the clinical examination of the challenging entity.

6.1.2 Systematic clinical examination

Factors to be evaluated clinically in food impactions include

- *Proximal contact between adjacent teeth*
- *Presence of proximal caries*
- *Approximation of contact areas in class II restorations*
- *Surface of proximal restorations whether polished or rough*
- *Shape of the embrasures*
- *Condition of interdental papilla*
- *Presence of gingival inflammation*
- *Probing depth in interdental region*
- *Presence of food debris or food particles*
- *Presence of calculus in the interdental region*

Once a thorough systematic clinical evaluation was executed, pertaining to initiating the management, a radiographic examination will be vital to validate the extent of periodontal involvement and to initiate a definitive treatment.

6.2 Radiographs as adjuvant

6.2.1 Intraoral periapical radiograph and bitewing radiograph

Radiograph acts as a necessary diagnostic tool to evaluate the extent and severity of periodontal lesions. Intraoral radiographs both intraoral periapical radiographs and bitewing radiographs are considered the most commonly used methods, which provide a two-dimensional view. A typical radiographic feature of food impaction exhibits complete loss of interdental bony crest, representing reverse bony architecture. It was empirical that bone quality and periodontal ligament space scored better on conventional intraoral radiography than CBCT. It was also evident that CBCT does not offer a significant advantage over conventional radiography for assessing periodontal bone levels [16].

6.2.2 CBCT

Various studies have reported that CBCT was as accurate as direct measurements using a periodontal probe and as reliable as intraoral radiographs for interproximal areas. 3D CBCT scanning has got advantages over periodontal probing and 2D intraoral radiography in assessing the exact amount of bone loss architecture. CBCT had better potential in detecting periodontal bone defects in all directions compared with periapical radiographs and was as reliable as radiographs for interproximal areas. CBCT could be considered a superior technique than conventional intraoral 2D radiography since the facial and lingual osseous defects could not be diagnosed with the 2D radiographs. Considering the various benefits, CBCT is currently being considered as a superior diagnostic tool for applications in periodontology [17, 18].

7. Management

7.1 Restorative

Proper proximal contact was crucial in maintaining functionality and stability of dental arch as well as periodontal health [19]. When restoring marginal ridges, deepening occlusal embrasure to provide adequate height helps create spillway for food to prevent vertical food impaction [4]. Cusp-marginal ridge occlusal contacts were predictive factors for contact failure in our specific sample. Periodic evaluation of dental restorations involving proximal surfaces with special attention to patient age and occlusal pattern are recommended. Stability of retreated defective restorations in patients with vertical food impaction was 66%–89% within a 10-year time frame [20].

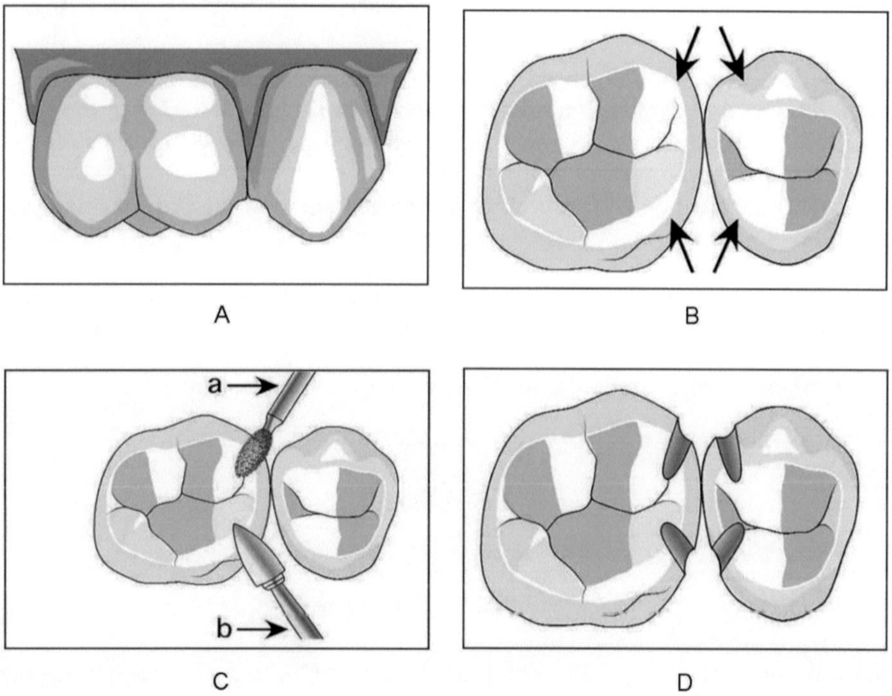

Figure 8.
A: no food escape grooves; B: points of preparation of escape grooves; C: grooves preparation using flame-shaped burs; D: final preparation of escape grooves.

7.1.1 Occlusal adjustment for food impaction

Patients with food impaction associated with a tight contact were evaluated for the presence of the following:

1. adequate food escape grooves

2. uneven marginal ridges

3. a prominent cusp opposing the contact area

When the food escape grooves were not noticed, one should prepare the food escape grooves in the the cuspal ridges just adjacent to the marginal ridges with a 5 mm long, 3.5 mm wide coarse, friction grip, football diamond stone (**Figure 8A–D**) [21]. If the marginal ridges were uneven, the more prominent ridge should be reduced. If a plunger cusp was detected, it should be reduced at the contact point while maintaining light occlusal contacts. All areas altered by the diamond stone were then smoothed with a 7 mm long, 2.5 mm wide friction grip, fine grit, flame-shaped, white Arkansas stone (**Figure 7a–d**) [21]. Care should be taken to remove a minimal amount of tooth structure or restoration to accomplish these goals.

7.2 Orthodontic correction

Among the factors, which contribute to localized periodontitis because of food, impaction is the malalignment of erupting teeth. The forceful wedging of food between the teeth during mastication occurs when proper contact relationship between approximating teeth.

Schuyler has stated definite objectives for correction of occlusal disharmony [22] including:

1. To associate the centric occlusion with unstrained maxilla-mandibular centric relation.

2. To obtain the maximum distribution of occlusal stress in centric relation.

3. To retain the maxilla-mandibular opening.

4. To equilibrate the steepness of similar tooth inclines, thereby distributing eccentric occlusal stresses.

5. To establish smoothness of guiding tooth inclines.

6. To minimize the incline of guiding tooth surfaces, so that occlusal stresses may more favourably be acting on the supporting tissues.

7. To retain the sharpness of cutting cusps.

8. To increase food exits.

9. To decrease contact surfaces.

Hence, it was clear that the role of an orthodontist is vital in evading periodontal disease caused by food impaction due to malocclusion by bringing out a harmonious occlusion to a dentition, which commonly acts as one of the predisposing factors.

7.3 Periodontal treatment

Hancock et al. [7] reported that 80% of proximal contacts with vertical food impaction had moderate-to-severe gingival inflammation (GI score >2). From this, it was evident that a significant proportion of patients with food impaction could be reported with periodontal problems. Therefore, a definitive periodontal treatment was obligatory for the patients with complaints of food impaction.

7.3.1 Phase I periodontal treatment

Phase I periodontal treatment is comprised of thorough scaling and root planning of the involved sites. The prime goal of nonsurgical periodontal treatment is to restore gingival health by completely removing the factors that provoke gingival inflammation (i.e., biofilm, calculus and endotoxin) from the tooth surface. A thorough scaling and root planning result in reduction of periodontal pathogens along with elimination of inflammation clinically [23].

Root surfaces with biofilm and calculus exposure stance a different problem of causing cemental irregularities [24]. Subgingival calculus was porous and harbours bacteria and endotoxin and therefore should be removed completely [25]. When dentin is exposed, biofilm bacteria may invade dentinal tubules. Therefore, scaling alone was insufficient to remove them, and a portion of the root surface must be removed to eliminate these deposits.

Patients with minimal amounts of calculus and relatively healthy periodontium can be treated in single appointment. Most other patients require multiple treatment sessions. The dentist should estimate the number of appointments needed on the basis of the number of involved teeth, severity of inflammation, amount and location of calculus, depth and activity of pockets, presence of furcation involvements and patient's compliance with oral hygiene maintenance.

It has been argued that such proficiency in instrumentation cannot be attained, and therefore periodontal surgery is necessary to gain access to root surfaces. Still, the mastery of scaling and root planning is essential to the ultimate success of any course of periodontal therapy.

Subgingival scaling and root planning are performed with universal or Gracey curettes by holding the curette with a modified pen grasp, the correct cutting edge slightly adapted to the tooth, with the lower shank kept parallel to the tooth surface and moved towards the tooth so that the face of the blade is nearly flush with the tooth surface. The blade was then inserted in the gingival sulcus and advanced to the base of the pocket using a light exploratory stroke. With a working angulation between 45 and 90 degrees, pressure is applied laterally against the tooth surface. Calculus is removed by short, powerful pull strokes (**Figure 9**). Once the calculus was removed, the resistance to the passage of the cutting edge of the curette diminishes until only a slight roughness remains. Longer, lighter root planning strokes are then activated with

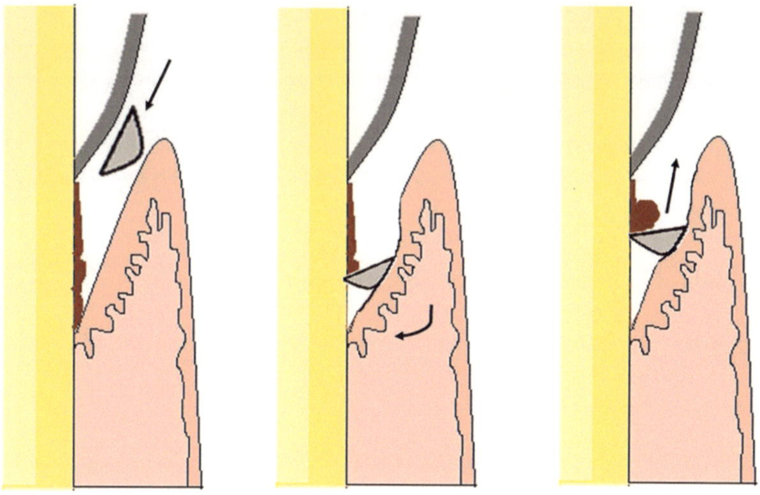

Figure 9.
Root surface planning using a curette with blade insertion and establishing stroke.

less lateral pressure until the surface of the roots is felt completely smooth without any irregularities [23].

7.3.2 Phase II periodontal treatment

Phase II periodontal treatment is performed only when the probing depth is 5 mm or greater, in accessible areas to perform scaling and root planning, lack of visibility to root surface, presence of subgingival calculus and its removal was difficult with scaling and root planning and evident bone loss.

Surgical periodontal therapy includes open flap debridement of the involved site using crevicular incision, full thickness flap reflection, thorough debridement of the site using curettes and/or ultrasonic scaler and then pacing the osseous defects using bone replacement grafts along with membrane over it and then approximating the flap using interrupted sutures.

Periodontal maintenance is vital following any means of periodontal management either phase I or phase II periodontal therapy.

7.3.3 Periodontal maintenance

Integrity of the proximal contact should be considered as primary factor for the periodontal maintenance of interproximal region. Each contact was tested twice with a double strand of unwaxed dental floss as described by O'Leary [26].

Each contact was described as given below:

1. Tight contact—definite resistance to the passage of dental floss.

2. Loose contact—minimal resistance to dental floss.

3. Open contact—no resistance to dental floss.

Based on the integrity of contact, need for creation of space between interdental contact areas to ease the entry of dental floss was established.

Based on the level of the presence of interdental papilla fill in the embrasure, oral hygiene maintenance, using various interdental cleansing aides, is to be prescribed for the patient (**Figure 10**).

1. No loss of interdental papilla: Dental floss

2. Interdental papilla loss of ½ the embrasure space: Interdental brush

3. Complete loss of interdental papilla: Uni-tuft brush

It was always pivotal to know that patients with evident interdental space, presence of interdental food impaction and loss of interdental papilla will have to rely on either of the interdental cleansing aides for their lifetime. Periodic review of the existing condition of interdental papilla health and interdental tooth or restorative surfaces with enforcement of scaling and root planning was central.

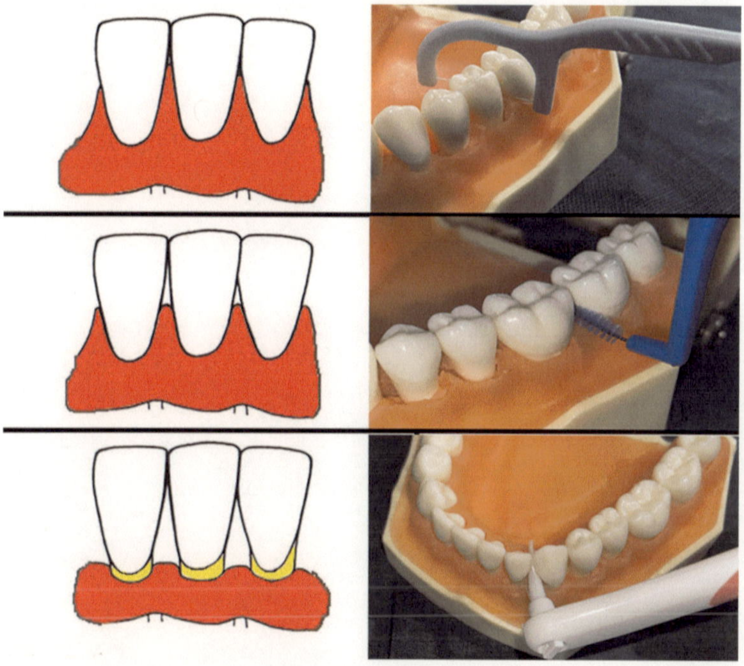

Figure 10.
Use of different interdental aides for different types of papilla.

8. Conclusion

Considering the aetiology as the fundamental core of food impaction, along with the aetiology, other factors, such as pattern of occlusion, periodontal status of the involved teeth and the harmonious alignment of the dentition, provided with the effective oral hygiene maintenance by the patient, plays a major role in the comprehensive management of the food impaction.

Acknowledgements

The authors would like to thank DH Newell, V John and S-J Kim for providing figures from their work to include in this chapter. The authors also extend thanks to Dr Mayur Khairnar for providing beautiful schematic representations of food impactions from his paper.

Conflict of interest

The authors declare no conflict of interest.

Author details

Renganath Murugan Jeyasree* and Thamilselvan Muthuraj
Department of Periodontics and Implantology, Rajas Dental College and Hospital, Tirunelveli, India

*Address all correspondence to: renganatharjun@gmail.com

References

[1] American Academy of Periodontology. Glossary of Periodontal Terms 2001. 4th ed. Chicago: American Academy of Periodontology; 2001

[2] Hirschfeld I. Food Impaction. Journal of American Dental Association. 1930;**17**: 1504

[3] Khairnar M. Classification of food impaction-revisited and its management. Indian Journal of Dental Advance. 2013; **5**(1):1113-1119

[4] Jung JH, Oh SC, Dong JK. A clinical study on the occurrence of food impaction. Journal of Korean Academy Prosthodont. 2000;**38**:50-58

[5] Gokhale S, Padmaja K. Food impaction after crown placements. Journal of Advanced Medicine. 2014; **2**(4):162-165

[6] Knezović Zlatarić D, Čelebić A, Valentić-Peruzović M. The effect of removable partial dentures on periodontal health of abutment and non-abutment teeth. Journal of Periodontology. 2002;**73**(2):137-144

[7] Hancock EB, Mayo CV, Schwab RR, Wirthlin MR. Influence of interdental contacts on periodontal status. Journal of Periodontology. 1980;**51**:445-449

[8] Jernberg GR, Bakdash MB, Keenan KM. Relationship between proximal tooth open contacts and periodontal disease. Journal of Periodontology. 1983;**54**(11):529-533

[9] Koori H, Morimoto K, Tsukiyama Y, Koyano K. Statistical analysis of the diachronic loss of interproximal contact between fixed implant prostheses and adjacent teeth. The International Journal of Prosthodontics. 2010;**23**:535-540

[10] Bidra AS. Nonsurgical management of inflammatory periimplant disease caused by food impaction: A clinical report. The Journal of Prosthetic Dentistry. 2014;**111**(2):96-100

[11] Maitland RI. Current concepts in successful posterior class II direct composites. Dental Economics. 1993;**83**: 101-103

[12] Nordho H, Leirskar J, von der Eehr FR. Saucer-shaped cavity preparations for posterior approximal resin composite restorations: Observations up to 10 years. Restorative Dentistry. 1998;**29**:5-11

[13] Raskin A, Michotte-Theall B, Vreven J, Wilson NHF. Clinical evaluation of a posterior composite 10-year report. Journal of Dental. 1999;**27**: 13-19

[14] Al-Anezi SA. The effect of orthodontic bands or tubes upon periodontal status during the initial phase of orthodontic treatment. The Saudi Dental Journal. 2015;**27**(3):120-124

[15] Levine S. The orthodontist, malocclusion and periodontal disease. Australian Orthodontic Journal. 1971; **2**(5):203-207

[16] AlJehani YA. Diagnostic applications of cone-beam CT for periodontal diseases. International Journal of Dentistry. 2014;**3**:2014

[17] Misch KA, Yi ES, Sarment DP. Accuracy of cone beam computed tomography for periodontal defect measurements. Journal of Periodontology. 2006;**77**(7):1261-1266

[18] Mol A, Balasundaram A. In vitro cone beam computed tomography imaging of periodontal bone. Dento

Maxillo Facial Radiology. 2008;**37**(6): 319-324

[19] Chow YC, Eber RM, Tsao YP, Shotwell JL, Wang HL. Factors associated with the appearance of gingival papillae. Journal of Clinical Periodontology. 2010;**37**:719-727

[20] Radafshar G, Khaghani F, Rahimpoor S, Shad A. Long-term stability of retreated defective restorations in patients with vertical food impaction. Journal of Indian Society Periodontology. 2020;**24**:329-333

[21] Newell DH, John V, Kim SJ, Harris RK. A technique of occlusal adjustment for food impaction in the presence of tight proximal contacts. Operative Dentistry. 2002;**27**(1):95-100

[22] Rothner JT. Occlusal equilibration—A part of orthodontic treatment. American Journal of Orthodontics. 1952; **38**(7):530-537

[23] Newman MG, Takei H, Klokkevold PR, Carranza FA. Newman and Carranza's Clinical Periodontology E-book. Elsevier Health Sciences; 2018

[24] Adriaens P, Edwards C, DeBoever J, et al. Ultrastructural observations on bacterial invasion in cementum and radicular dentin of periodontally diseased human teeth. Journal of Periodontology. 1988;**59**:493

[25] Cadosch J, Zimmermann U, Ruppert M, et al. Root surface debridement and endotoxin removal. Journal of Periodontal Research. 2003;**38**:229

[26] O'Leary TJ, Badell MC, Bloomer RS. Interproximal contact and marginal ridge relationships in periodontally healthy young males classified as to orthodontic status. Journal of Periodontology. 1975;**46**(1):6-9

Chapter 4

The Two-Way Relationship between Diabetes Mellitus and Periodontal Disease: A New Insight

Leela Subhashini C. Alluri, Kristen Puckett, Chethan Sampath, David A. Mott, Kaitlyn Logan, Jazmyne Walker, Gerald Davis, Cherae Farmer-Dixon and Pandu R. Gangula

Abstract

Periodontal Disease and Diabetes Mellitus are two chronic systemic diseases that are intimately connected. A bidirectional relationship exists between the two; to study this unique relationship, they must be studied separately as independent malfunctions and in tandem. Patients that experience these conditions exhibit similar innate immune responses, which lead to aggravated dysfunction of specific body systems. In patients where both conditions exist simultaneously, Diabetes and Periodontal Disease can act in a synchronistic manner, worsening symptoms. In this chapter, the epidemiology of the diabetes mellitus and periodontal disease, presence of biomarkers have been reviewed, and the metabolic syndrome, clinical relevance and treatment modalities, complications of diabetes mellitus, and guidelines for the general dentists, primary care physician, periodontist have been discussed.

Keywords: diabetes mellitus, biomarkers, periodontitis, periodontal disease, type one diabetes mellitus, type two diabetes mellitus

1. Introduction

The epidemiologic relationship between Diabetes Mellitus Type I and II (TIDM and TIIDM, respectively) and Periodontitis is well documented and multifaceted. Diabetes is a widespread disease estimated to affect 415 million adults, 20–79 years of age, with many remaining undiagnosed with approximately 193 million. Further, half a million children aged 14 and under live with Type 1 Diabetes Mellitus (TIDM). Additionally, 318 million adults are believed to have some form of glucose intolerance, placing them into the "pre-diabetic" category and increasing their risk of eventually developing the disease. TIDM and TIIDM caused 5 million deaths in 2015, accumulating a financial burden of between USD 673 billion and USD 1197 billion in healthcare spending. If this rise is not slowed, it is estimated that by the year 2040, there will be 642 million people living with diabetes [1]. There exists a large pool of evidence for the association between periodontitis and TIIDM, and the bidirectional nature of the relationship is well established [2]. In turn, people with TIIDM exhibit decreased glycemic control. Further studies must examine the association between periodontitis and TIDM. In TIDM, an immune cascade results in the beta cells of the pancreas being attacked, decreasing insulin secretion. TIDM only accounts for approximately 10% of all diabetic patients [3]. In a small percentage of these patients, there is no β cell destruction, making the pathogenesis idiopathic [4]. TIIDM is a systemic metabolic disease in which there is insulin resistance or defective in insulin secretion or a combination of both. The number of people living with Diabetes Mellitus has nearly quadrupled in the last four decades [5].

Periodontal disease (PD) affects 47.2% of adults aged 30 years and older, and the incidence of developing some form of periodontal disease increases with age, with 70.1% of adults aged 65 and older having periodontal disease [6]. Periodontal disease affects men more than women, with the incidence rates being 56.4% and 38.4%, respectively. Socioeconomic factors also play a role, with 65.4% of individuals affected living below the poverty line and 66.9% of those without a high school education [6]. In addition, smoking plays a factor, with 64.2% of current smokers developing periodontal disease [6]. The pathogenesis of periodontal disease is well studied and understood. The interaction between periodontal pathogenic microorganisms and the host immune system leads to the secretion of proinflammatory cytokines, which leads to the destruction of the periodontium compromising the affected tooth prognosis [7].

2. Detection of the presence of type 2 diabetes mellitus and periodontitis using biological markers

Periodontitis has been intricately linked to TIDM and TIIDM in various documented studies, showing that uncontrolled diabetes can initiate and promote the progression of periodontal disease. In return, periodontitis can decrease in insulin secretion leading to hyperglycemic state and the risk for further complications [5]. Therefore, early detection of both these diseases is of the utmost importance. Clinically, diagnosing periodontitis via clinical attachment level, periodontal probing depth, bleeding on probing, and radiographic evidence of bone loss are implemented and true methods; however, early detection using biological markers such as salivary proteins can be beneficial to earlier management of periodontitis. Levels of inflammatory chemokines such as interleukin (IL)-6 and tumor necrosis factor-alpha (TNF-α) increase in the case of PD; thus, these are used in studies as biological markers along with IL-1β, interleukin-6 (IL-6), and several macrophage molecules such as macrophage inflammatory protein (MIP)-1α and matrix metalloproteinase-8 (MMP-8) [8]. The primary functions of these cytokines in the body are an increased immune response and systemic inflammation, which further causes decrease in insulin secretion or insulin resistance in diabetic patients [8]. In addition, lipopolysaccharide (LPS) from the surface membrane of Gram-negative bacteria in the oral cavity can trigger the production of proinflammatory cytokines. Thus, increasing the number of pathogenic Gram-negative bacteria in the oral cavity can further exacerbate local and systemic inflammation.

One advantage of using biomolecules for detecting periodontitis in diabetic patients is the non-invasive nature of detection and earlier intervention. Salivary concentrations of IL-1β, IL-6, and macrophage inflammatory protein (MIP)-1α can be easily sampled from gingival crevicular fluid, and quantitative analysis is performed via fluorescent immunoassay. A study published by Miller et al. in 2020 demonstrated that several biomarkers could yield greater specificity for the detection of periodontitis [8]. This provides promising results for early detection and diagnosis. The study also concluded that MMP-8 and IL-1β present in the gingival crevicular fluid (GCF) could discriminate periodontitis in patients with TIIDM [8]. MMP-8 has been studied extensively as a biomarker for periodontal disease, and meta-analysis studies have shown it to be both practical and a promising biomolecule for more accurate early diagnosis in the near future [9].

Another useful biological marker that can be utilized for the detection of both periodontal disease and TIIDM is the hormone somatostatin. The autoregulation of somatostatin receptor 2 in periodontal cells has been studied under several conditions, including inflammatory and specific obesity-related conditions. Immunocytochemistry, a study method in which antibodies are used as markers to test for antigens, is utilized in these studies, such as these and polymerase chain reactions to replicate and better view DNA fragments. There is significant upregulation in somatostatin receptor 2 in periodontal ligament cells, including osteoblasts, osteoclasts, odontoblasts, cementoblasts, fibroblasts, and undifferentiated mesenchymal cells when exposed to proinflammatory molecules [8]. In addition, Leptin and visfatin are adipokines that have been studied, and both exist at heightened levels in obese patients [8]. These adipokines are marked and studied in patients with periodontitis and can be quantitatively measured in the gingival crevicular fluid [10]. In the presence of periodontal disease, leptin and visfatin exist at heightened levels, suggesting an increase in local and systemic production.

2.1 Interleukin-1 biomarker

IL-1β is a key mediator of the host inflammatory response, and it increases damage at the cellular and tissue level during times of chronic disease, which is of particular interest in patients with existing periodontal disease. IL-1β is the most studied IL-1 family, and no signal sequence is required for IL-1β secretion; instead, it employs several non-conventional pathways rather than conventional protein secretion [11]. This is favorable for study and why IL-1β is such an effective biomarker for periodontitis analysis. The IL-1 family of cytokines contributes to leukocyte migration and relocation, stimulating osteoblasts and resulting in bone resorption, which is vital for longitudinal periodontitis study. A study conducted by Kornman et al. found that non-smoking, healthy patients with altered IL-1β alleles indicative of a positive genotype showed a risk of developing chronic periodontitis up to seven times compared to the baseline [12]. This cornerstone study opened other studies focusing on the IL-1 family and utilizing cytokines as biological markers for periodontal disease and other proinflammatory diseases such as TIIDM and metabolic disorders.

Interleukin-1 genotypes were explored more thoroughly in a study by Brodzikowska et al., in which the presence of two specific polymorphisms of IL-1 was observed in vivo to determine whether severe periodontitis has a genetic factor [13]. IL-1β is released into the oral environment and displays agonistic action upon receptor binding [13]. IL-1α and IL-1β are located on the "q" arm of chromosome 2 – the human chromosome that provides instructions for making proteins. Differences in the amount of IL-1 secretion in response to microbial infection may contribute to differences in risk for periodontitis and the severity of the disease [13]. This distinction is in allele 2 on chromosome 2, the substitution of nucleotide thymine for cytosine [13]. Like the study cited above, this study also concludes that in individuals with this allele substitution, periodontitis is seven times more likely to develop [13]. Without simultaneous substitution of alleles, patients instead developed moderate periodontitis compared to severe when both alleles are present, demonstrating that genetic factors play a role in not only the development of the disease but the severity as well [13].

2.2 C-reactive protein (CRP)

C-reactive protein (CRP) is a biological marker that is highly sensitive and nonspecific, making it an ideal biomarker. It is produced in the liver in response to systemic and local injury or trauma. Certain conditions have been shown to increase levels of CRP, including but not limited to pregnancy, smoking, and obesity [14]. CRP also exists at heightened levels in the body after the production of interleukins, such as IL-1α and IL-1β, as mentioned previously in this chapter. CRP is considered a risk factor for developing TIIDM and cardiovascular disease [14]. CRP has also been studied regarding periodontitis, though sparingly. In one study, Esteves-Lima et al. showed that a heightened level of CRP contributes to higher rates of periodontitis, and this further demonstrates the systemic impact that periodontitis has on the body [14].

Interestingly, the presence of *Porphyromonas gingivalis,* a Gram-negative pathogenic bacterium, increases CRP levels in 20% of patients [14]. Whether the levels of CRP can be quantified and extrapolated to the severity of the periodontal disease is slightly debated. One study by Torrungruang et al. shows promising results that increased levels of CRP are directly correlated to the severity of periodontal disease; for every 1 mm increase in periodontal probing depth or clinical attachment loss, the odds of having sST2, a serum cardiac biomarker like CRP, in increased by 70% and 30%, respectively [15]. Biomarkers help in detection, earlier intervention, and managing periodontal disease and diabetes mellitus.

3. The bidirectional relationship between type 2 diabetes mellitus, periodontal disease, and obesity: a metabolic syndrome

3.1 Periodontal disease and obesity

Periodontal disease is defined as chronic, progressive destruction of the periodontium. Obesity is a chronic metabolic disease, which increases the risk of developing various other medical conditions, such as atherosclerosis, hypertension, TIIDM, and cardiovascular disease. In addition, obesity is a risk factor for periodontitis [16]. Statistically significant changes in histology of periodontium have been observed in cases of hereditary obesity [14]. The link between obesity and periodontal disease has been studied as well, with alveolar bone resorption rate being higher in obese rats as compared to non-obese animals [14]. Excess body fat accumulation causes metabolic syndromes and diseases, the most notable being insulin resistance, high triglycerides, low levels of HDL (High-Density Lipoprotein), nonalcoholic fatty liver disease (NAFLD), β cell dysfunction in the pancreas, and TIIDM. Research has shown that periodontitis is correlated with insulin resistance and increased systemic inflammation. Periodontitis, obesity, and TIIDM all have similar pathogenic pathways. Body fat distribution has been demonstrated to play a role in the development of TIIDM and periodontitis. Visceral adipose tissue is metabolically more active than subcutaneous adipose tissue, in addition to secreting higher levels of adipocytokines than subcutaneous adipose tissue [17]. Because adipose tissue secretes proinflammatory cytokines such as adipocytokines, there is a higher chance of insulin resistance developing, which further causes infiltration of proinflammatory macrophages and an increase in plasma free fatty acids (FFAs) [18]. Huang et al. demonstrated that periodontal pathogen-derived virulence factors such as lipopolysaccharide (LPS) and palmitate (major saturated fatty acid) upregulated periodontal expression of free fatty acid receptors (GPR40 and CD36) in obese and TIIDM patients [17]. Systematic reviews strongly suggest a physiologic association between periodontitis, obesity, and type 2 diabetes mellitus. In addition, there is an association between obesity and periodontal disease regarding health behaviors such as inactivity. Obesity can contribute to a chronic systemic inflammatory state, producing malignant microflora in the oral cavity that promotes inflammatory pathways [18]. Studies have also shown that increased gingival index and periodontal pocket depths are associated with increased triglyceride levels and low HDL [19].

3.2 Periodontal disease and diabetes mellitus

Diabetes is a multifaceted chronic, systemic disease involving decreased insulin secretion, peripheral tissues resistant to insulin, or a combination of both. The effects of periodontal disease on glycemic control demonstrate that diabetes mellitus and periodontal disease have a bidirectional relationship [20] (**Figure 1**).

Individuals with existing diabetes increase the risk of developing periodontal diseases, and patients with comorbidities such as diabetes and periodontal diseases develop poor glycemic control and rapid progression of the periodontal disease. To understand the effects of periodontal disease, the advanced glycated end products (AGE)-receptors of AGE (RAGE) pathway must be explained [4]. The AGE-RAGE signaling pathway is a cascade feed-forward loop, AGE interacts with RAGE present on the immune, endothelial, and epithelial cells, this phenomenon results in increased

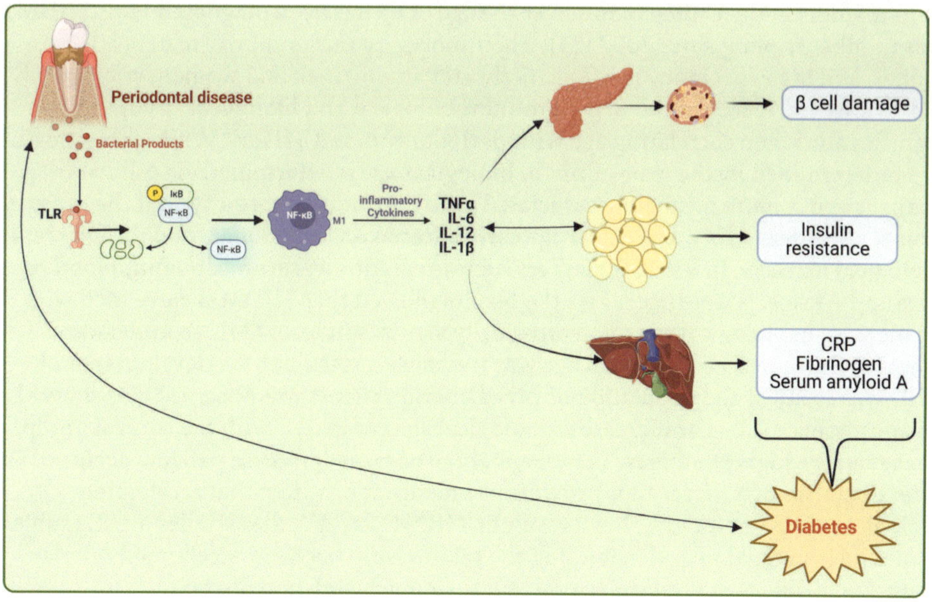

Figure 1.
The bidirectional and pathophysiological mechanisms involved in periodontal and TIIDM. The figure is created with BioRender©.

oxidative stress, increased RAGE expression (due to the forward-feedback loop), and pro-inflammatory cytokines lead to cell and tissue damage.

There exists a bidirectional relationship between diabetes and periodontal disease, with one influencing another and sometimes exhibiting overlapping physiological patterns and symptoms. In one 2-year longitudinal study, patients with diabetes (TIDM and TTDM) and severe periodontitis were at a sixfold higher risk of poor glycemic control [4]. Effective treatment in the periodontally diseased patient can significantly improve the metabolic function of TIDM and TIIDM patients. After the periodontal intervention, such as scaling and root planning, glycosylated hemoglobin (HbA1c) levels in people with diabetes decreased. In a meta-analysis, periodontal therapy, and appropriate maintenance intervals (3 and 6 months) caused a statistically significant reduction in HbA1c [21]. Furthermore, periodontal treatment with a 1-year follow-up examination was administered to patients with periodontal disease, and diabetes results showed a statistically significant amount of decreased gingival crevicular fluid biomarkers from baseline to 12 months compared with untreated patients with periodontal disease [22]. Patients also had a 0.6% decrease in HbA1c score post-treatment [22]. This further shows the dynamic relationship between the two diseases and how systemic inflammation can be reduced through the treatment of periodontal disease, and that this should be a core component of diabetes care.

3.3 The bidirectional relationship between type 2 diabetes mellitus and periodontal disease: age and gender -related factors

The bidirectional relationship between TIIDM and periodontitis is established. However, other factors such as BMI (Body Mass Index), age, and smoking status must also be considered. Age is one factor that significantly contributes to both TIIDM and periodontal disease. With advancing age comes higher susceptibility to microbial infections due to higher levels of Gram-negative bacteria in the oral cavity [19]. One in four adults in the United States over the age of 65 has been diagnosed with TIIDM, this number tripling since 2007 [23]. Their mortality risk is approximately 50% higher, and life expectancy is 5–7 years shorter among men and women, respectively [24]. However, it is essential to note the chronological and biological age difference significantly when correlating age with periodontitis and TIIDM. While chronologic age is determined by the time of birth, biological age is determined via cellular changes and is more intimately associated with morbidity, mortality, and the progression of the disease [24]. Biological age can be traced on the cellular level using several biological markers. In a study, markers such as creatinine, serum albumin, blood pressure and A1c levels were used, and the results showed that TIIDM is correlated with an increase in biological age on a statistically significant level [24]. To understand whether the increased biological age was the cause or result of the development of TIIDM, a study of the population of pre-diabetic patients was observed and showed an approximate 2.7-year increase in biological age compared with the control group. However, the highest increase in biological age observed in these patients occurred after diagnosis of TIIDM, thus providing evidence for the fact that accelerated biological age is not a cause, but a result of TIIDM [24]. Further studies on this subject would be beneficial to understanding the relationship between accelerated cellular aging and diabetes as it relates to oral and systemic health and disease.

There is something to be said about gender -related factors when it comes to both periodontal disease and obesity. Female patients that go through pre- and post-menstrual phases have higher induction of proinflammatory cytokines in the periodontium, which can cause an increased risk of periodontitis [25]. In one study by Estevez-Lima et al., the incidence of women developing TIIDM with a previous medical history of gestational diabetes was observed at approximately 18%, and the incidence of periodontitis was approximately 10% [14]. The way in which the body handles renal glucose also has a gender -related component, and since this plays a significant role in HbA1c levels, which in turn has implications for periodontal disease severity, it must be discussed. Studies also show that women are less likely to develop TIIDM and periodontitis, although they are more likely than men to develop diabetic comorbidities such as cardiovascular and end-stage renal disease [26].

3.4 The bidirectional relationship between type 2 diabetes mellitus and periodontal disease: lifestyle habits

According to the latest National Institute of Health data (2021), adult obesity affects approximately 16 of the world's population. Behavioral patterns play a significant role in this. A cross-sectional study by Khan et al. in 2020 explored the relationship between behavioral change that reduces systemic inflammation and the reduction of periodontitis risk [16]. The results of this study suggested that the effect of TIIDM on periodontitis is higher than the effect of obesity on periodontitis [16]. This demonstrates that confounding variables exist when exploring the relationship between diabetes mellitus and periodontitis and that further studies demonstrating causality should be performed. Somatostatins, interleukins, and adipokines have been discussed previously in this chapter as biological markers for studying both diabetes and periodontal disease. In addition, several members of the IL-6 family exist at elevated levels in patients with periodontitis [17]. The prevalence of periodontitis was 97% in patients with obesity, and approximately 60% of these obese patients had mild to moderate periodontitis (CPI score 3.) An additional 38% of patients studied had a CPI score of 4, indicating severe periodontitis [25].

Interestingly, in this study, the prevalence of periodontitis was significantly higher in patients in the middle age range compared to younger obese adults. Aging and periodontal disease are closely related, as there is a cumulative periodontal tissue and alveolar bone breakdown with age [25]. This is compounded by aging, increasing body fat, and decreasing lean protein mass and bone mineral density.

4. Clinical relevance and treatment modalities

Improving glucose control may be key to preventing complications of TIIDM and chronic periodontitis [27, 28]. Metformin, a second-generation biguanide, is a medication that assists in blood glucose level control. It decreases glucose absorption by the small intestine and increases the body's sensitivity to insulin. In one study, differing percentages of metformin gel were applied in the periodontal pockets of participants, as well as a placebo gel for control [29]. Local delivery of Metformin gel stimulates a significant increase in probing depth reduction [29]. Local treatment of metformin in the periodontal pocket can be enhanced with biological aids such as the drug delivery carrier polylactic-co-glycolic acid (PLGA) [30]. In-vitro bioavailability is significantly improved with PLGA, and when drug efficacy is increased, treatment is enhanced, and prognosis improves. PLGA simultaneously increases the concentration of Metformin at the action site and decreases the concentration at non-target sites [30]. When the clinical efficacy of Metformin was studied, a significant reduction in pocket depth and increase in clinical attachment level were observed, and results still showed an improvement in periodontal health [31]. This evidence suggests the importance of using biological aids such as Metformin as an adjunct therapy to traditional treatments such as SRP (Scaling and Root Planing) [31]. The use of local drug delivery into the periodontal pockets is traditional; systemic antimicrobials such as minocycline, doxycycline, chlorhexidine, and tetracycline have been used in patients with periodontal disease [31]. Recently, adjuvant antibiotic therapy has been studied on periodontal patients with diabetes.

TIDM and TIIDM are considered risk factors for periodontitis due to the increased risk of systemic infection, collagen synthesis impairment, and impairment of glycosaminoglycan by gingival fibroblasts [32]. In addition, collagen breakdown and the gingival crevicular fluid are increased. Adjunctive therapy may improve the efficacy of SRP in reducing probing depth in patients with diabetes. Local drug delivery directly into the periodontal pockets is an example of adjunct therapy on the rise due to its promising clinical results. SRP with ozone gas therapy as an adjunct constituent can reduce Hb1Ac levels in diabetic patients [33]. Poor response to traditional periodontal treatment, such as scaling and root planning, is associated with an increased risk (37%) of developing TIIDM in the future [29]. Regardless of treatment modality, the treatment of periodontal disease, in general, improves the overall metabolic health of those patients with TIDM and TIIDM. Non-surgical periodontal therapy, such as SRP, improves general health for patients with TIIDM [34].

Periodontal treatment in a diabetic patient can help improve glycemic control. At least seven randomized clinical trials and four systemic meta-analyses have demonstrated that there is a clinically significant reduction in glycosylated hemoglobin levels in TIIDM diabetes patients [35, 36]. The results from these studies showed a decrease between 0.27 and 0.48% 3–4 months post-periodontal therapy. More research must be conducted to demonstrate that this positive result is consistent after 6 months or more post-treatment. Improvements in glycosylated hemoglobin levels are consistent with the magnitude of increase in HbA1c levels experienced by diabetic patients with periodontitis, an average of 0.29% [36]. Therefore, there is a remarkably similar inverse relationship between the rise in HbA1C attributed to periodontitis in the diabetic patient and the fall in HbA1C levels after the periodontal intervention. Periodontal therapy and appropriate maintenance intervals can help diabetic patients with short-term glycemic control. In the other direction, examining the periodontitis patient regarding diabetes, severe periodontal disease is strongly associated with elevated Hb1AC levels. In patients diagnosed with diabetes, hyperglycemia was observed, and in patients without diabetes, there was still an increase in Hb1AC, the difference being a lower serum level [37]. There is also a direct correlation between the severity of periodontal disease and the severity of cardiovascular and nephrotic complications [38]. Elevated lipid levels and elevated oxidative stress markers exist in the serum of TIIDM patients [39]. New evidence also demonstrates that people with severe periodontitis have an increased risk of developing TIIDM [40–42]. Meta-analyses provide abundant evidence for improved glycemic control in the TIIDM patient after periodontal treatment for up to 3 months. One systematic review showed a mean reduction of 0.36% 3 months after periodontal treatment [35].

There is a continuous global research effort on the bidirectional relationship between periodontitis and diabetes. This abundance of evidence-based information allows the medical team, including physicians, to follow specific guidelines to better manage diabetic/periodontal patients and their overall health. A workshop conducted by the European Federation of Periodontology (EFP) and the International Diabetes Federation (IDF) in 2012 provided guidelines for the treatment and management of these patients, resulting in consensus statements and intervention treatments to be followed by oral healthcare workers and the medical team [43]. Among people who have not been diagnosed with diabetes, periodontitis is still associated with increased blood glucose levels. Patients with periodontitis alone have higher fasting glucose levels when compared to periodontally healthy patients [44]. Because of this, periodontal patients exhibit a higher chance of developing pre-diabetes or diabetes [44]. In diabetic patients, cytokines and other biomarkers play a role in the pathogenesis of periodontitis. Elevated levels of pro-inflammatory mediators such as TNF- α, IL-1, and IL-6 exist in the periodontal pocket in uncontrolled or poorly controlled diabetes patients. Cell cultures exposed to high glucose levels display the destruction of hard and soft tissues; therefore, high glucose levels in the oral cavity in people with diabetes play a significant role in destroying the periodontium [45]. Short-term (3–6 months) periodontal intervention reduces HbA1C levels, similarly, to adding another antidiabetic medication to the patient's regimen. If this can be extrapolated past 6 months of periodontal treatment with further studies, it would have positive implications for reducing diabetes-associated morbidity and mortality rates.

5. Complications of diabetes

The complications of diabetes include cardiovascular diseases, end-stage renal disease, retinopathy, nephropathy, neuropathy, and neuropathic foot ulcers. Periodontitis is the sixth most complication in diabetic patients. These comorbidities

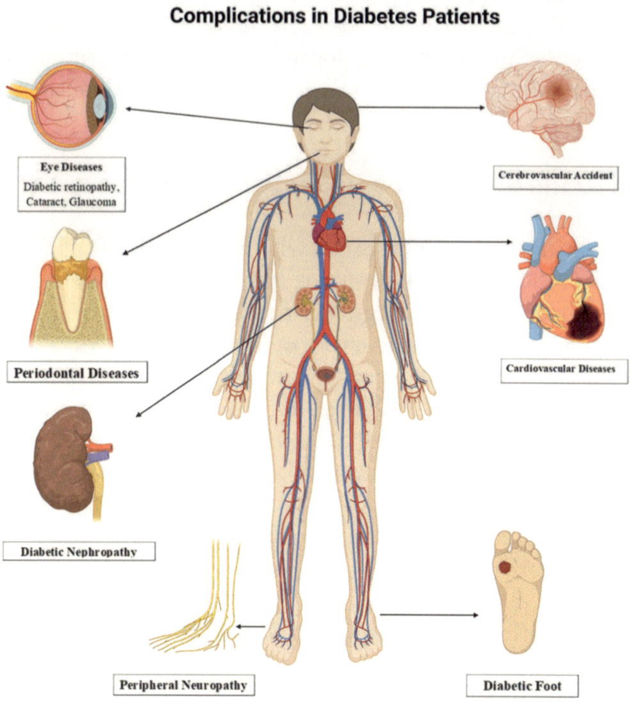

Figure 2.
Complications in uncontrolled diabetic patients. The figure is created with BioRender©.

have been studied extensively among 34,149 study subjects through meta-analysis and have been adjusted for confounding variables. In patients with comorbid periodontitis and diabetes, retinopathy is significantly increased, and severity is directly proportional to the severity of the periodontal disease. Further, evidence from three studies demonstrates more renal complications in patients with either TIDM or TIIDM and periodontitis. In one study, chronic kidney disease was found to be strongly associated with cardiovascular disease when both diabetes and periodontal disease were present in the patient, compared with patients with only one of the comorbidities [46]. Periodontal patients exhibiting severe periodontitis (in conjunction with diabetes) have an increased incidence of foot ulcerations. There is a demonstratable association between patients with TIIDM and periodontitis and several cardiovascular conditions, including cardiovascular mortality, coronary heart disease, cerebrovascular accidents, and heart disease. Overall, mortality is significantly increased in patients with both TIIDM and periodontitis and is well documented in the literature. **Figure 2** explains the macrovascular and microvascular complications in uncontrolled diabetic patients.

6. Guidelines for the medical team

The dental team and other medical professionals must know the signs of periodontal disease and its link to poor glycemic control. Pre-diabetes and undiagnosed diabetes can be managed better through early intervention by the entire medical team. Guidelines should be followed to minimize the negative impacts of chronic, systemic pathogenesis associated with periodontal disease and diabetes. Since there is an increased risk of developing periodontitis in the diabetic patient and, in turn, negative complications associated with periodontitis and glycemic control, the following guidelines are recommendations for physicians and dentists alike [1]:

7. Recommendations for the general dentist and periodontist

- Patients presenting to the dental office without a diagnosis of diabetes with an increased risk for TIIDM should be educated about their risk level and referred to a physician for appropriate diagnosis if signs are present. These signs can be evaluated using a medical history form, questionnaire, or screening based upon the guidelines of the American Diabetes Association. Symptoms that are observed, such as polydipsia, polyuria, and polyphagia, should be referred to a physician for an evaluation immediately. Before the patient is dismissed, they should be well educated on periodontitis and how to take preventative measures.

- Patients should be informed that lifelong maintenance is required for periodontitis, and personalized care should be given depending on the patient's periodontal status.

- Oral health instructions are to be provided at every appointment with diabetic patients. Examples of individualized care include brushing twice a day, flossing, and using specific dentifrices and mouth rinses.

- Patients should be informed that if periodontitis is left untreated, tooth loss may occur, and glycemic control will be more challenging to manage. Even if symptoms are not worsening, the disease can still progress. Because of this, regular dental visits and adherence to a maintenance schedule must occur.

- Diabetic patients should be informed that they are at an increased risk of developing the periodontal disease compared to non-diabetic patients and that untreated periodontitis can negatively impact metabolism and increase the risk of developing systemic health complications.

- Diabetic patients should be educated on prognosis after periodontal therapy and how it can have positive implications for metabolic control and lessening complications of diabetes.

- Diabetic patients should be informed that conditions such as xerostomia (dry mouth) and burning mouth syndrome can develop, as well as an increased incidence of oral fungal infections such as candidiasis.

- If after intraoral examination no periodontitis is diagnosed, patients with diabetes should be placed on preventative care and regularly monitored for any changes in their oral health.

- If periodontitis is diagnosed, they should undergo treatment immediately, regardless of diabetes control, as non-surgical periodontal therapy can help improve glycemic control.

- If the patient in question does have a positive history of periodontitis, re-evaluation of the periodontium is recommended before each annual appointment [1].

8. Recommendations for the primary care provider

- The medical team should conduct a thorough medical history to determine whether the patient has TIDM or TIIDM and the presence of existing complications.

- All patients recently diagnosed with TIDM or TIIDM should be referred for a periodontal examination. Even if periodontal disease is not detected, an annual examination is recommended.

- Children under 17 years of age diagnosed with TIDM or TIIDM should undergo annual periodontitis screening by a dentist.

- Diabetic patients who have experienced tooth loss are encouraged to seek appropriate dental treatment to maintain masticatory function and adequate nutrition.

- Diabetic patients should be informed that wound healing can be impaired or take longer than patients without diabetes.

- The physician and dental team should discuss diabetes management before oral evaluation and treatment to prevent a hypoglycemic incident.

- Physicians should inquire about whether diabetic patients have had a previous periodontal diagnosis and whether they are undergoing periodontal maintenance.

- Diabetic patients (TIDM and TIIDM) should be advised at every annual appointment in the primary practitioner's office that they are at an increased risk of gingivitis and periodontitis. These conditions should be explained accordingly so that the patient is well-informed on which signs and symptoms to look for. Glycemic control should be discussed in relation to periodontal disease, explaining how H1Ac control can be more challenging when periodontitis is present.

- Medications the patient is taking, such as anticoagulant drugs or lipid-lowering agents, should be considered when doing a medical evaluation, as this can impact periodontal treatment.

- The physician/primary care provider should ask when the patient's last blood glucose levels had been checked and request that they bring a copy of this result to their appointment.

- Oral health education and instructions should be provided to all diabetic patients in all medical settings, including individualized advice on the management of an appropriate oral hygiene route antimicrobial mouthwash, and TIIDM patients should undergo a thorough oral examination by the dental team, including full-mouth periodontal pocket charting and bleeding scores if indicated [1].

9. Conclusions

Dentists often focus on treating the periodontium and dentition rather than overall health of the patient. This chapter highlights the fallacy in this approach and reminds dental specialists that systemic diseases such as Type 2 Diabetes Mellitus and Periodontal Disease are often comorbid and should be treated as such. Several therapies discussed are improving, and several loom on the horizon, promising to improve both periodontal health and the overall health of the patient. Therapies such as traditional, non-surgical intervention and local delivery of Metformin provide promising results for both periodontal and systemic health.

Conflict of interest

The authors declare no conflict of interest.

Author details

Leela Subhashini C. Alluri[1*], Kristen Puckett[2], Chethan Sampath[3], David A. Mott[1], Kaitlyn Logan[4], Jazmyne Walker[4], Gerald Davis[2], Cherae Farmer-Dixon[5] and Pandu R. Gangula[3]

1 Department of Periodontics, Meharry Medical College, Nashville, TN, USA

2 Department of Restorative, Meharry Medical College, Nashville, TN, USA

3 Department of ODS and Research, Meharry Medical College, Nashville, TN, USA

4 Meharry Medical College, Nashville, TN, USA

5 Department of Dental Public Health, Meharry Medical College, Nashville, TN, USA

*Address all correspondence to: lalluri@mmc.edu

References

[1] Sanz M et al. Scientific evidence on the links between periodontal diseases and diabetes: Consensus report and guidelines of the joint workshop on periodontal diseases and diabetes by the International Diabetes Federation and the European Federation of Periodontology. Diabetes Research and Clinical Practice. 2018;**137**:231-241

[2] Taylor GW. Bidirectional interrelationships between diabetes and periodontal diseases: An epidemiologic perspective. Annals of periodontology. Dec 2001;**6**(1):99-112

[3] Mobasseri M et al. Prevalence and incidence of type 1 diabetes in the world: A systematic review and meta-analysis. Health Promotion Perspectives. 2020;**10**(2):98

[4] Kay A, Simpson C, Stewart J Jr. The role of AGE/RAGE signaling in diabetes-mediated vascular calcification. Journal of Diabetes Research. Oct 2016;**2016**

[5] Wu C-Z et al. Epidemiologic relationship between periodontitis and type 2 diabetes mellitus. BMC Oral Health. Dec 2020;**20**(1):1-15

[6] Eke PI et al. Advances in surveillance of periodontitis: The Centers for Disease Control and Prevention periodontal disease surveillance project. Journal of Periodontology. 2012;**83**(11):1337-1342

[7] Rahim MI et al. Bacterial-specific induction of inflammatory cytokines significantly decreases upon dual species infections of implant materials with periodontal pathogens in a mouse model. Biomedicines. 26 Jan 2022;**10**(2):286

[8] Miller CS et al. Salivary biomarkers for discriminating periodontitis in the presence of diabetes. Journal of Clinical Periodontology. Feb 2021;**48**(2):216-225

[9] Gul SS et al. Efficacy of MMP-8 level in gingival crevicular fluid to predict the outcome of nonsurgical periodontal treatment: A systematic review. International Journal of Environmental Research and Public Health. 7 Mar 2022;**19**(5):3131

[10] Deschner J et al. The role of adipokines in periodontal infection and healing. Molecular oral microbiology. Dec 2014;**29**(6):258-269

[11] Memmert S et al. Regulation of somatostatin receptor 2 by proinflammatory, microbial and obesity-related signals in periodontal cells and tissues. Head and Face Medicine. Dec 2019;**15**(1):1-9

[12] Kornman KS et al. The interleukin-1 genotype as a severity factor in adult periodontal disease. Journal of Clinical Periodontology. Jan 1997;**24**(1):72-77

[13] Brodzikowska A, Górska R, Kowalski JJA. Interleukin-1 genotype in periodontitis. Archivum Immunologiae et Therapiae Experimentalis. Dec 2019;**67**(6):367-373

[14] Esteves-Lima R-P et al. Association between periodontitis and serum c-reactive protein levels. Journal of Clinical and Experimental Dentistry. Sep 2020;**12**(9):e838

[15] Torrungruang K et al. Periodontitis is associated with elevated serum levels of cardiac biomarkers—Soluble ST2 and C-reactive protein. Journal of Clinical Periodontology. Aug 2019;**46**(8):809-818

[16] Khan MS et al. Obesity and periodontal disease: A review. Journal of Family Medicine and Primary Care. Jun 2020;**9**(6):2650

[17] Li G et al. Upregulation of free fatty acid receptors in periodontal tissues of patients with metabolic syndrome and periodontitis. Journal of Periodontal Research. Aug 2019;**54**(4):356-363

[18] Khan S et al. Association between obesity and periodontitis in Australian adults: A single mediation analysis. Journal of Periodontology. Apr 2021;**92**(4):514-523

[19] Ngoude JXE et al. Relationship between periodontal diseases and newly-diagnosed metabolic syndrome components in a sub-Saharan population: A cross sectional study. BMC Oral Health. Dec 2021;**21**(1):1-7

[20] Teshome A, Yitayeh AJB. The effect of periodontal therapy on glycemic control and fasting plasma glucose level in type 2 diabetic patients: Systematic review and meta-analysis. BMC Oral Health. Dec 2017;**17**(1):1-11

[21] Chen Y-F et al. Baseline HbA1c level influences the effect of periodontal therapy on glycemic control in people with type 2 diabetes and periodontitis: A systematic review on randomized controlled trails. Diabetes Therapy. May 2021;**12**(5):1249-1278

[22] Preshaw PM et al. Treatment of periodontitis reduces systemic inflammation in type 2 diabetes. Journal of Clinical Periodontology. Jun 2020;**47**(6):737-746

[23] Genco RJ, Borgnakke WSJP. Risk factors for periodontal disease. Periodontology. 2013;**62**(1):59-94

[24] Bahour N et al. Diabetes mellitus correlates with increased biological age as indicated by clinical biomarkers. GeroScience. Feb 2022;**44**(1):415-427

[25] Alsalihi L et al. Prevalence of periodontitis in obese patients in Bahrain: A cross-sectional study. BMC Oral Health. 2021;**21**(1):1-8

[26] Major RW et al. The kidney failure risk equation for prediction of end stage renal disease in UK primary care: An external validation and clinical impact projection cohort study. PLoS medicine. 6 Nov 2019;**16**(11):e1002955

[27] Barutta F et al. Novel insight into the mechanisms of the bidirectional relationship between diabetes and periodontitis. Biomedicines. 16 Jan 2022;**10**(1):178

[28] Iwashita M et al. The link between periodontal inflammation and obesity. Current Oral Health Reports. 1 Oct 2021:1-8

[29] Pradeep A et al. Efficacy of varying concentrations of subgingivally delivered metformin in the treatment of chronic periodontitis: A randomized controlled clinical trial. Journal of Periodontology. Feb 2013;**84**(2):212-220

[30] Pereira ASBF et al. In vitro-in vivo availability of metformin hydrochloride-PLGA nanoparticles in diabetic rats in a periodontal disease experimental model. Pharmaceutical Biology. 1 Jan 2021;**59**(1):1574-1582

[31] Patil KS et al. Efficacy of 1.5% metformin gel as an adjuvant to scaling, root planing, and curettage for the treatment of infrabony defects in chronic periodontitis patients. Contemporary Clinical Dentistry. Jan 2022;**13**(1):18

[32] Grellmann AP et al. Systemic antimicrobials adjuvant to periodontal therapy in diabetic subjects: A

meta-analysis. Journal of Clinical Periodontology. Mar 2016;**43**(3):250-260

[33] Rapone B et al. The effect of gaseous ozone therapy in conjunction with periodontal treatment on glycated hemoglobin level in subjects with Type 2 diabetes mellitus: An unmasked randomized controlled trial. International Journal of Environmental Research and Public Health. Aug 2020;**17**(15):5467

[34] Quintero AJ et al. Effect of two periodontal treatment modalities in patients with uncontrolled type 2 diabetes mellitus: A randomized clinical trial. Journal of Clinical Periodontology. Sep 2018;**45**(9):1098-1106

[35] Engebretson S, Kocher TJJ. Evidence that periodontal treatment improves diabetes outcomes: A systematic review and meta-analysis. Journal of Clinical Periodontology. Apr 2013;**40**:S153-S163

[36] Madianos PN, Koromantzos PAJJ. An update of the evidence on the potential impact of periodontal therapy on diabetes outcomes. Journal of Clinical Periodontology. Feb 2018;**45**(2):188-195

[37] Borgnakke WS et al. Effect of periodontal disease on diabetes: Systematic review of epidemiologic observational evidence. Journal of Periodontology. Apr 2013;**84**:S135-S152

[38] Zardawi F et al. Association between periodontal disease and atherosclerotic cardiovascular diseases: Revisited. Frontiers in Cardiovascular Medicine. 15 Jan 2021;7:625579

[39] Allen EM et al. Oxidative and inflammatory status in Type 2 diabetes patients with periodontitis. Journal of Clinical Periodontology. Oct 2011;**38**(10):894-901

[40] Demmer RT, Jacobs DR Jr, Desvarieux MJD. Periodontal disease and incident type 2 diabetes: Results from the First National Health and Nutrition Examination Survey and its epidemiologic follow-up study. Diabetes Care. 1 Jul 2008;**31**(7):1373-1379

[41] Morita I et al. Relationship between periodontal status and levels of glycated hemoglobin. Journal of Dental Research. Feb 2012;**91**(2):161-166

[42] Saito T et al. The severity of periodontal disease is associated with the development of glucose intolerance in non-diabetics: The Hisayama study. Journal of Dental Research. Jun 2004;**83**(6):485-490

[43] Chapple IL, Genco R. Periodontology, Diabetes and periodontal diseases: Consensus report of the Joint EFP/AAP Workshop on Periodontitis and Systemic Diseases. Journal of Periodontology. Apr 2013;**84**:S106-S112

[44] Graziani F et al. A systematic review and meta-analysis of epidemiologic observational evidence on the effect of periodontitis on diabetes an update of the EFP-AAP review. Journal of Clinical Periodontology. Feb 2018;**45**(2):167-187

[45] Polak D, Shapira LJJ. An update on the evidence for pathogenic mechanisms that may link periodontitis and diabetes. Journal of Clinical Periodontology. Feb 2018;**45**(2):150-166

[46] Sharma P et al. Association between periodontitis and mortality in stages 3-5 chronic kidney disease: NHANES III and linked mortality study. Journal of Clinical Periodontology. Feb 2016;**43**(2):104-113

Chapter 5

"Interleukin" – An Essential Mediator of the Pathophysiology of Periodontitis

Avishek Das and Debajyoti Mondal

Abstract

Chronic periodontitis is a multifactorial polymicrobial disease caused by a complex interaction between periodontal pathogens and host immune response. This interaction is largely regulalated by a group of signaling molecules called Interleukins. Initially, investigators believed that interleukins were made chiefly by leukocytes to act primarily on other leukocytes, and for this reason they named them interleukins, meaning "between leukocytes". The majority of interleukins are synthesized by helper CD4+ T lymphocytes, as well as through monocytes, macrophages, and endothelial cells. Interleukins provide information to various inflammatory cells to produce essential proteins which exert pro inflammatory as well as anti inflammatory responses. This chapter will emphasize the role of interleukins in the pathophysiology of periodontitis.

Keywords: periodontitis, interleukins, genetic polymorphism, transcription factors, modulation of signaling, mRNA stability

1. Introduction

Interleukins are a group of cytokines (secreted proteins/signaling molecules) that are expressed by white blood cells. Initially, investigators believed that interleukins were made chiefly by leukocytes to act primarily on other leukocytes, and for this reason they named them interleukins, meaning "between leukocytes". The majority of interleukins are synthesized by helper CD4+ T lymphocytes, as well as through monocytes, macrophages, and endothelial cells. In 1977, **Steve Gillis & Kendal A. Smith** found that *T cell Growth Factor (TCGF)* is needed by Cytotoxic T Lymphocyte Lines to kill leukemia cells [1]. In 1979, it was found that *Lymphocyte Activating Factor (LAF)* produced by macrophages could enhance the production of TCGF. So LAF name was changed to *Interleukin-1* because it functioned first in the sequence and TCGF became *IL-2* because it came second though it was the first interleukin to be discovered. Interleukins are broadly classified as pro- inflammatory (IL -1, IL-6, IL-8, IL-17) and anti-inflammatory (IL-4, IL-6, IL-10, IL-11, IL-13, IL- 16). Though there are many interleukins, which exerts dual action.

2. Pro-inflammatory interleukins

2.1 Interleukin-1

The original members of the IL-1 superfamily are IL-1α, IL-1β and the IL-1 Receptor antagonist (IL-1RA). IL-1α and -1β are pro-inflammatory cytokines. The receptors for interleukin 1 are Interleukin 1 receptor, type I (IL-1RI) and Interleukin 1 receptor, type II (IL-1RII). IL-1R1 found in astrocytes, chondrocytes, keratinocytes, oocytes, fibroblasts etc. IL-1α binds preferentially to IL-1RI. IL-1RII found in B cells, T cells, keratinocytes, monocytes and neutrophils. IL-1β binds to IL-1RII. Besides the above two there is *IL-1RI accessory protein (IL-1RAcP)* which is a transmembrane glycoprotein. It interacts with *IL-1RI* only, but shows no affinity for IL-1α, IL-1β or IL-1receptor antagonist. IL-1α ligation of the type 1 IL-1 receptor (IL-1R1) leads to multiple pro inflammatory effects [2], including cytokine secretion, neutrophil recruitment, and upregulation of major histocompatibility complex (MHC) and co stimulatory molecules on antigen presenting cells. Pro-IL-1α (p33) is processed to mature IL-1α (p17) by calpain [3] and it increases its affinity for IL-1 Receptor I. IL-1 receptor 2 (IL-1R2) whose binding to pro-IL-1α inhibited its cytokine activity. IL-1α also has powerful effects on adaptive immunity by enhancing expansion and survival of T cells, differentiation of **T helper 17 (Th17) cells**, and effector T cell proliferation in the presence of **regulatory T cells** [4]. IL-1β is a pro-inflammatory cytokine. Although little or no IL-1ß is normally detected in human plasma or serum obtained from healthy, rested human subjects, elevated levels have been reported in the circulation of febrile or septic patients, in patients with inflammatory disease like chronic periodontitis. IL-1RA is a molecule that competes for receptor binding with IL-1α and IL-1β thus blocking their role in immune activation. Interleukin 1 receptor antagonist is used in the treatment of rheumatoid arthritis and diabetes mellitus. Its commercial variety ANAKINRA blocks Interleukin-1 (which causes impaired insulin secretion, decreased cell proliferation and apoptosis in patients with type 2 diabetes mellitus) and thus improves glycemic and pancreatic beta cell secretory function.

2.2 Interleukin-6

IL-6 increases the synthesis of the two major acute-phase proteins, *C-reactive protein (CRP),* which increases the rate of phagocytosis of bacteria, and *serum amyloid A (SAA)* by regulating changes in the gene transcription rate of these proteins. It also increases the synthesis of fibrinogen. Interleukin-6 is especially important in the early stages of T-cell differentiation. In this phase, it reinforces the effect of IL-2 and promotes the differentiation of CD4 cells into T-helper2 cells [5]. IL-6 enhances the release of antibodies by acting as a growth factor for already differentiated plasma cells. It stimulates mostly the release of IgG from these cells [6].

2.3 Interleukin-8

Interleukin-8 (IL-8) is a chemokine produced by macrophages, epithelial cells and endothelial cell. IL-8 was renamed CXCL8 by the Chemokine Nomenclature Subcommittee of the International Union of Immunological Societies. IL-8's primary function is to recruit neutrophils to phagocytose the antigen which trigger the antigen pattern toll-like receptors. It serves as a chemical signal that attracts neutrophils at the site of inflammation, and therefore is also known as a *neutrophil chemotactic factor*.

2.4 Interleukin-17

It is also a pro inflammatory cytokine produced by T- helper cells. To elicit its function,IL-17 binds to type 1 cell surface receptor called IL-17R of which there are 3 variants IL-17RA, IL-17RB and IL-17RC. IL-17 inhibits the gingival endothelial cell expression of developmental endothelial locus-1(DEL-1) which is an endogenous inhibitor of neutrophil adhesion dependent on LFA-1 and ICAM-1 ligation [7].

2.5 Genetic polymorphism of pro-inflammatory interleukins

Kornman et al. first reported on polymorphism for IL-1 genes in relation to chronic periodontitis. IL-1β in GCF was 2.5 times higher in patients showing genetic polymorphism at IL-1α-889 and IL-1β + 3954 (IL-1 composite genotype). Even in these sites after treatment, IL-1β in GCF was still 2.2 times higher for IL-1 composite genotype patients [8]. *N Sharma et al in 2014* demonstrated the association of genetic polymorphism of IL-6 [−597/−174] with chronic periodontitis [9]. *Zacarias et al in 2015* showed that IL-17A G197A rs 2,275,913 polymorphism, AA genotype and A allele could be associated with the susceptibility to chronic periodontitis [10]. Das et al. 2021 suggested a strong association of polymorphism of IL-12β (rs7709212) in both chronic and aggressive periodontitis in a group of the Bengali population [11].

3. Anti-inflammatory interleukins

Pro-inflammatory interleukins induce a Th1, pro-inflammatory phenotype in lymphocytes, while anti-inflammatory interleukins induce a shift to a Th2 profile, with attenuation of pro-inflammatory cytokine expression and concomitant increase in anti-inflammatory cytokine expression.

3.1 Interleukin-10 [IL-10]

is considered a prototype anti-inflammatory cytokine. Its effector functions include a shift of T cell cytokine expression from a Th1 to a Th2 profile, and attenuation of the production of pro-inflammatory cytokines.

3.2 Interleukin-4 (IL-4)

Promotes a Th2 response in lymphocytes and it also negatively regulates the production of pro-inflammatory cytokines [12].

3.3 Interleukin-19

Has been recently described [2000] IL-10 family member and shares 20% amino acid identity to IL-10. It decreases the expression of IFNγ and increases the expression of IL-4 in T lymphocytes [13].

3.4 Molecular mechanism of anti-inflammatory interleukins

The molecular mechanism of anti-inflammatory interleukins can be categorized into the following categories:

3.4.1 Modulation of signaling

The specificity of signaling between different interleukins often lies with different, specific usage of "cytokine-specific" STAT(signal transducer and activator of transcription) proteins. The IL-10 activity requires STAT3, which transactivates multiple genes germane to regulation of the inflammatory response, and STAT3 is required for IL-10 attenuation of TNFα induced inflammatory events. IL-10 binding to IL-10 receptor activates the IL-10/JAK1/STAT3 cascade, where phosphorylated STAT3 homodimers translocate to the nucleus within seconds to activate the expression of target genes. Upon entering the nucleus, STAT3 activates specific target genes among which the ultimate effectors of the ANTI-INFLAMMATORY RESPONSE (the 'AIR factors') are found. STAT3's role is to stimulate the expression of specific genes (AIR factors), which in turn suppress the expression of pro-inflammatory genes. STAT6 is an IL-4–induced transcription factor, and it was reasoned that this factor might block NF-κB activation by binding it directly and/or by preventing its DNA binding activity. STAT6 is required for IL-4 inhibition of osteoclastogenesis [14]. Anti-inflammatory cytokines have also evolved the capacity to diminish Mitogen Activated Protein Kinase [MAPK] signaling.

3.4.2 Modulation of transcription factors

A second mechanism whereby anti-inflammatory interleukins exert their effects is by modulation of NF-κB activity. The NF-κB complex is a cytoplasmic transcription factor consisting of 2 subunits (p50 and p65). NF-κB is present in the cytoplasm, where it exists in an inactive form. Upon stimulation with inflammatory factors, an inhibitory protein termed IκB disassociates from this complex and is proteolyticaly degraded, allowing the p50/p65 complex to translocate into the nucleus and act as a transcriptional activator. NF-κB is considered to be a "**master switch**" in transactivation of multiple genes involved in the inflammatory response.IL-4 can negatively regulate NF-κB by increasing **IκB** transcription, leading to increased binding and inhibition of NF-κB nuclear translocation [14]. Correspondingly, both IL-10 and IL-13 can also reduce or prevent IκB degradation. IL-10 can target other transcription factors as well like Early growth response factor-1 (Egr-1). It has been found that IL-10 can significantly decrease Lipopolysaccharide (LPS) stimulated Egr-1 activation in macrophages, indicating a more direct link to inhibition of proliferation [15].

3.4.3 Regulation of gene expression and mRNA stability

Anti-inflammatory interleukins can also prevent inflammatory response by destabilization of mRNA transcripts mediated by mRNA-binding stability factors [16]. The 3′ untranslated region (UTR) of many transcripts associated with inflammation contain an AU-rich elements (AREs) which are target sites for these mRNAs-binding stability factors. Up regulation of one of these mRNAs stability factors, **HuR** (a ubiquitously expressed member of the Hu family of RNA-binding proteins), can support hyper activation of inflammatory mediators. One manuscript describes the down-regulation of HuR by IL-10 in monocytes and attributes this as a major mechanism whereby IL-10 exerts systemic anti-Inflammatory effects [17].

3.5 Relationship between anti-inflammatory interleukins and statins

Several studies demonstrate that Statins can inhibit MAPKs, including p44/42 and p38, and can directly modulate inflammatory gene expression by diminishing activity of NF-κB [18]. In T cells, statins can also induce the release of Th2 promoting cytokines, including IL-10, and diminish secretion of Th1 cytokines such as IL-2 [19].

3.6 Genetic polymorphism of anti-inflammatory interleukins

Dong CHEN et al. in 2016 did one study aimed to evaluate whether three single nucleotide polymorphisms (SNPs), rs2070874 and rs2243248 from *IL4* and rs1800925 from *IL13*, are associated with chronic periodontitis in a Han Chinese population consisting of 440 moderate or severe CP patients and 324 healthy controls [20]. Zahra Armingohar et al. in 2015 studied seventy-two patients with vascular disease(VD)of whom 35 had Chronic Periodontitis were genotyped for single nucleotide polymorphisms (SNPs) in the IL10 – 592 (rs1800872), –819 (rs1800871), and – 1082 (rs1800896) gene by Taqman rtPCR method and by DNA sequencing [21]. The C alleles and C/C genotypes of IL10 – 592 and IL10 – 819 frequencies were significantly higher, while the frequencies of the IL10 – 592 (C/A) and IL10 – 819 (C/T) heterozygote genotypes were significantly lower in the VD group with CP compared to those without chronic periodontitis. The IL10 haplotype ATA frequency (–1082, –819, –592) showed a trend to a significant difference between the two groups indicating protection against chronic periodontitis.

4. Role of interleukins in the inflammatory process of periodontitis

The inflammatory process of periodontitis is initiated by the activation of specific protein structures called Toll-like receptors (TLRs) situated on the wall of the epithelial cells of the sulcular epithelium [22]. The function of these TLRs is to recognize the lipoproteins and peptidoglycans of gram positive bacteria (TLR-2) and lipopolysaccarides of gram negative bacteria (TLR-4) [23]. The recognition of bacterial substances through TLRs of epithelial cells leads to the activation of cell mediated immune response which is regulated by subsets of CD4 + T cells called T helper (Th) cells. The different subsets of T helper cells are characterized by releasing different cytokine profiles.Th-1 cells are mainly responsible for the secretion of pro-inflammatory interleukins (IL-1, IL-2, IL-12), while Th-2 cells induces the release of anti-inflammatory interleukins (IL-4, IL-5, IL-6, IL-10, IL-13) [24]. Apart from this Th-17 cells release IL-17 which helps in rapid neutrophil recruitment during early stage of the inflammatory process of periodontitis [25]. Interleukin-8 or CXCL8 establishes a chemotactic gradient for this neutrophil emigration.

The persistent presence virulent factors within the subgingival microenvironent leads to shift of the cellular profile from polymorphonuclear leukocyte to mononuclear leukocyte.IL-6 plays major role in shifting of this cellular profile. There are two types of IL-6 receptors, membrane bound receptors present on the wall of PMNLs(mIL-6R) and soluble receptors present freely in extravascular spaces (sIL-6R). Large number of neutrophils which are migrated during early stages of inflammatory process cleave their mIL-6R from cell membrane to inhibit further binding with IL-6. Thus the free receptors easily coupled with IL-6 and this complex further attaches with gp-130 subunit situated on the endothelial cell membrane. This leads to release of monocyte chemoattractant protein –1 (MCP-1) which creates a chemotactic gradient for the transmigration of monocytes [5].

IL-1, IL-6 and TNF-α induces the differentiation of these recruited monocytes into preosteoclasts [26].

5. Therapeutic strategies for the potential use of interleukin blockage in periodontitis

The benefit of IL-1 blockage has been demonstrated in conditions, such as gout, diabetes mellitus and even myeloma [27]. Studies have discussed that blocking of IL-1 may reduce the periodontal bone loss and also suggesting future prospects [28].

Anakinra (Kineret) was the first interleukin-1 blocking agent to get the approval for the treatment of rheumatoid arthritis in the USA in 2001. It is a recombinant IL-1 receptor antagonist. However, due to short half-life (4–6 h) daily subcutaneous injections were required [29]. In comparison to Anakinra, other agents like **Rilonacept** (recombinant soluble receptor which prevents IL-1β to bind to membrane bound receptors presents on the cell membrane of inflammatory cells, thus inhibits further signal transduction) and **Canakinumab** (monoclonal antibody against IL-1β) have longer half life. Rilonacept has a half life of 6–8 days,while the half life of canakinumabis as long as 26 days [29, 30].

6. Inflammasome inhibitors

NLRP3 inflammasome helps in the maturation of IL-1β. Inflammasome inhibitors target caspas-1 and NLRP3,thus prevents the maturation of IL-1β. **Belnacasan** (VX-765, Vertex Pharmaceuticals) a caspas-1 inhibitor partly decreases bone resorption in the periapical lesion of rat experimental apical periodontitis [31].

7. Conclusion

Hence interleukins can be considered as the group of signaling molecules that provide information to various inflammatory cells to produce essential proteins which exerts pro inflammatory as well as anti inflammatory responses. They also play crucial role in shifting of polynuclear to mononuclear cellular profile and further differentiation of pro bone resorptive cells. Therapeutic strategies of blocking Interleukin functions through receptor antagonist, soluble receptors, monoclonal antibodies and inflammasome inhibitors showed beneficial outcomes. However, more investigation is necessary for interleukin blockage to be used as a treatment for periodontitis or as an adjunctive to periodontal therapy.

Author details

Avishek Das* and Debajyoti Mondal
Dr R Ahmed Dental College and Hospital, Kolkata, India

*Address all correspondence to: avidoc2010@gmail.com

References

[1] Gillis S, Smith K. Long term culture of tumour-specific cytotoxic T cells. Nature. 1977;**268**:154-156. DOI: 10.1038/268154a0

[2] Dinarello CA. Immunological and inflammatory functions of the interleukin-1 family. Annual Review of Immunology. 2009;**27**:519-550. DOI: 10.1146

[3] Kobayashi Y, Yamamoto K, Saido T, Kawasaki H, Oppenheim JJ, Matsushima K. Identification of calcium-activated neutral protease as a processing enzyme of human interleukin 1 alpha. Proceedings of the National Academy of Sciences of the United States of America. 1990;**87**:5548-5552

[4] Sims JE, Smith DE. The IL-1 family: Regulators of immunity. Nature Reviews. Immunology. 2010;**10**(2):89-102. DOI: 10.1038/nri2691

[5] Janeway CA Jr, Travers P, Walport M, et al. Immunobiology: The Immune System in Health and Disease. 5th ed. New York: Garland Science; 2001. Available from: https://www.ncbi.nlm.nih.gov/books/NBK10757

[6] Maeda K, Mehta H, Drevets DA, Coggeshall KM. IL-6 increases B-cell IgG production in a feed-forward proinflammatory mechanism to skew hematopoiesis and elevate myeloid production. Blood. 2010;**115**(23):4699-4706. DOI: 10.1182/blood-2009-07-230631

[7] Eskan MA, Jotwani R, Abe T, et al. The leukocyte integrin antagonist Del-1 inhibits IL-17-mediated inflammatory bone loss. Nature Immunology. 2012;**13**(5):465-473. Published 2012 Mar 25. DOI: 10.1038/ni.2260

[8] Kornman KS, Crane A, Wang HY, di Giovine FS, Newman MG, Pirk FW, et al. The interleukin-1 genotype as a severity factor in adult periodontal disease. Journal of Clinical Periodontology. 1997;**24**(1):72-77. DOI: 10.1111/j.1600-051x.1997.tb01187.x

[9] Sharma N, Joseph R, Arun R, Radhakrishnan C, Srinivas L, Banerjee M. Cytokine gene polymorphism (interleukin-1β +3954, Interleukin-6 [−597/−174] and tumor necrosis factor-α-308) in chronic periodontitis with and without type 2 diabetes mellitus. Indian Journal of Dental Research. 2014;**25**:375-380. DOI: 10.4103/0970-9290.138343

[10] Zacarias JMV, Sippert EÂ, Tsuneto PY, Visentainer JEL, Silva CDO e, Sell AM. The influence of interleukin *17A* and *IL17F* polymorphisms on chronic periodontitis disease in brazilian patients. Mediators of Inflammation. 2015;**2015**:8. DOI: 10.1155/2015/147056

[11] Das A, Pal A, Bagchi S. Genetic polymorphism of interleukin-12β (rs7709212) in chronic and aggressive periodontitis in a group of the Bengali population of India. Journal of Global Oral Health. 2021;**4**:78-83

[12] Urban JF Jr, Katona IM, Paul WE, Finkelman FD. Interleukin 4 is important in protective immunity to a gastrointestinal nematode infection in mice. Proceedings of the National Academy of Sciences of the United States of America. 1991;**88**(13):5513-5517. DOI: 10.1073/pnas.88.13.5513

[13] Jordan WJ, Eskdale J, Boniotto M, Lennon GP, Peat J, Campbell JD, et al. Human IL-19 regulates immunity through auto-induction of IL-19 and

production of IL-10. European Journal of Immunology. 2005;**35**(5):1576-1582

[14] Abu-Amer Y. IL-4 abrogates osteoclastogenesis through STAT6-dependent inhibition of NF-kappaB. The Journal of Clinical Investigation. 2001;**107**(11):1375-1385. DOI: 10.1172/JCI10530

[15] Kamimura M, Viedt C, Dalpke A, Rosenfeld ME, Mackman N, Cohen DM, et al. Interleukin-10 suppresses tissue factor expression in lipopolysaccharide-stimulated macrophages via inhibition of Egr-1 and a serum response element/MEK-ERK1/2 pathway. Circulation Research. 2005;**97**(4):305-313

[16] Katsanou V, Papadaki O, Milatos S, Blackshear PJ, Anderson P, Kollias G, et al. HuR as a negative posttranscriptional modulator in inflammation. Molecular Cell. 2005;**19**(6):777-789. DOI: 10.1016/j.molcel.2005.08.007

[17] Rajasingh J, Bord E, Luedemann C, Asai J, Hamada H, Thorne T, et al. IL-10-induced TNF-alpha Mrna destabilization is mediated via IL-10 suppression of p38 MAP kinase activation and inhibition of HuR expression. The FASEB Journal. 2006;**20**(12):2112-2114

[18] Huang KC, Chen CW, Chen JC, Lin WW. Statins induce suppressor of cytokine 24 neurismal-3 in macrophages. FEBS Letters. 2003;**555**(2):385-389

[19] Dunn SE, Youssef S, Goldstein MJ, Prod'homme T, Weber MS, Zamvil SS, et al. Isoprenoids determine Th1/Th2 fate in pathogenic T cells, providing a mechanism of modulation of autoimmunity by atorvastatin. The Journal of Experimental Medicine. 2006;**203**(2):401-412

[20] Dong C, Zhang T-l, Wang X. Association between polymorphisms in interleukins 4 and 13 genes and chronic periodontitis in a han chinese population. BioMed Research International. 2016;**2016**:7. DOI: 10.1155/2016/8389020

[21] Armingohar Z, Jørgensen JJ, Kristoffersen AK, Schenck K, Dembic Z. Polymorphisms in the interleukin-10 gene and chronic periodontitis in patients with atherosclerotic and aortic 26 neurismal vascular diseases. Journal of Oral Microbiology. 2015;7:26051. DOI: 10.3402/jom.v7.26051

[22] Song B, Zhang YL, Chen LJ, et al. The role of toll-like receptors in periodontitis. Oral Diseases. 2017;**23**(2):168-180

[23] Ford PJ, Gamonal J, Seymour GJ. Immunological differences and similarities between chronic periodontitis and aggressive periodontitis. Periodontology 2000. 2010;**53**(1):111-123

[24] Mosmann TR, Sad S. The expanding universe of T-cell subsets: Th1, Th2 and more. Immunology Today. 1996;**17**(3):138-146

[25] Harrington LE, Hatton RD, Mangan PR, et al. Interleukin 17-producing CD4+ effector T cells develop via a lineage distinct from the T helper type 1 and 2 lineages. Nature Immunology. 2005;**6**(11):1123-1132

[26] Cochran DL. Inflammation and bone loss in periodontal disease. Journal of Periodontology. 2008;**79** (8 Suppl):1569-1576

[27] Dinarello CA. An expanding role for interleukin-1 blockade from gout to cancer. Molecular Medicine. 2014;**20**:S43-S58

[28] Assuma R, Oates T, Cochran D, Amar S, Graves DT. IL-1 and TNF antagonists inhibit the inflammatory

response and bone loss in experimental periodontitis. Journal of Immunology. 1998;**160**:403-409

[29] Arranz L, Arriero MDM, Villatoro A. Interleukin-1beta as emerging therapeutic target in hematological malignancies and potentially in their complications. Blood Reviews. 2017;**31**:306-317

[30] Grom AA, Horne A, De Benedetti F. Macrophage activation syndrome in the era of biologic therapy. Nature Reviews. Immunology. 2016;**12**:259-268

[31] Cheng R et al. The extent of pyroptosis varies in different stages of apical periodontitis. Biochimica et Biophysica Acta. 2018;**1864**:226-237

Chapter 6

Role of Cellular Responses in Periodontal Tissue Destruction

Nam Cong-Nhat Huynh

Abstract

Periodontal tissue destruction is the deterioration of tooth-supporting components, particularly the periodontal ligament (PDL) and alveolar bone, resulting in gingival recession, root exposure, tooth mobility and drifting, and, finally, tooth loss. The breakdown of the epithelial barriers by infection or mechanical damage allows bacteria and their toxins to enter and stimulates the immune response. The bacteria cause periodontal damage via the cascade of the host reaction which is crucial in the destruction of the connective tissue around the tooth. The OPG/RANKL/RANK system is the key player in bone regulation of periodontal tissue and was controlled by both immune and non-immune cells. This knowledge has predicated the successfulness of implant and orthodontics treatments with the predictable healing and regeneration of the bone and supporting tissues surrounding the teeth.

Keywords: RANKL, OPG, RANK, osteoimmunology, periodontal destruction, periodontitis, bone resorption, inflammation, immune response

1. Introduction

The periodontium is made up of four components: gingiva, alveolar bone, cementum, and periodontal ligament (PDL) (**Figure 1**) [1]. They differ in cellular composition, protein kinds and quantities, mineralization, metabolic activity, and disease susceptibility. Embryologically, the gingival component is produced from the pharyngeal arches' ectoderm and contains stratified squamous epithelium while PDL, cementum, and alveolar bone are produced from neuro-mesenchymal stem cells and contain connective tissues [2]. Periodontal destruction is initiated by bacterial agents (periodontitis) or mechanism stimuli (such as orthodontic force or dental trauma). However, host response plays a very important role in the demolition of the connective tissue around the tooth. In this chapter, we concisely discussed the cellular responses, including immune and non-immune cells to the destruction of periodontal tissue, and how we applied the knowledge in dental practice.

2. Periodontal tissues destruction

The components of periodontal tissue can be divided into hard tissue (cementum and alveolar bone) and soft tissue (gingiva and PDL). The anchors to which the

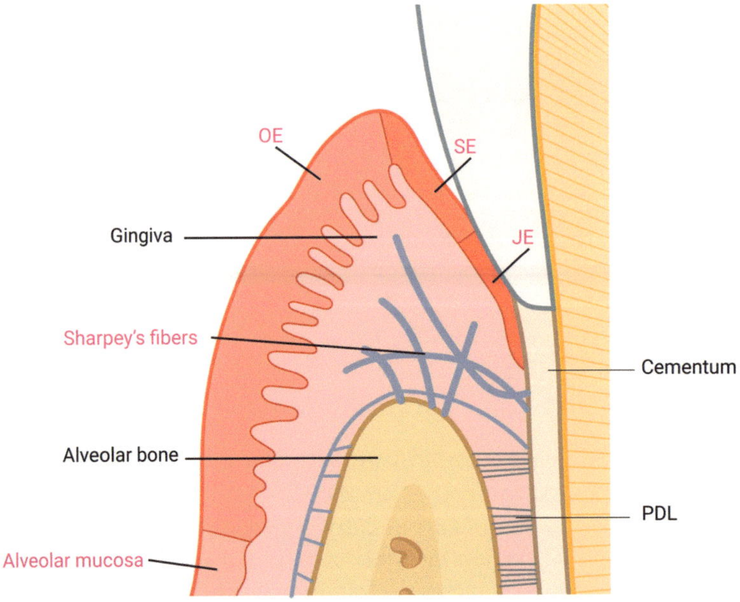

Figure 1.
Periodontium is made up of four components: gingiva, alveolar bone, cementum, and periodontal ligament (PDL). Oral epithelium (OE): is the epithelium that exposes to the surface of the mouth. Sulcular epithelium (SE): is the epithelium that contacts the surface of the tooth. Paroxizmalnaya form epithelium (JE): the epithelium which connects the gingiva to the tooth. OE, SE, and JE are keratinized tissue while alveolar mucosa is non-keratinized. Created with BioRender.com.

fibrous PDL binds the tooth into the skeleton are the two mineralized tissues, cementum and alveolar bone [3]. The gingiva is the periodontium's covering tissue, providing immediate protection for the underlying tissues and extra tooth attachment. The cementum is the calcified avascular mesenchymal tissue that forms the anatomic root's outer layer. The periodontium's primary roles include protecting teeth, nerves, and blood vessels from mechanical stresses, attaching teeth to the bone, and transmitting occlusal forces and sensibility to stimuli such as temperature and pain [4].

Periodontitis (PD) is a common illness that can lead to tooth loss and causes a slew of problems for physicians. Periodontitis is caused by inflammation of the tooth-supporting tissues, which results in the gradual loss of PDL and alveolar bones [5]. Periodontal disease is a collection of chronic inflammatory diseases that affect the gingiva, bone, and ligament (the connective tissue collagen fibers that bind a tooth to the alveolar bone) that support the teeth [6]. Chronic periodontitis occurs when untreated gingivitis progresses to the loss of gingiva, bone, and ligament, resulting in the deep periodontal 'pockets' that are a characteristic of the condition and can eventually lead to tooth loss. Periodontal disease can aggravate inflammatory illnesses, such as diabetes and atherosclerosis by increasing the body's total inflammatory load.

On the other hand, apical periodontitis (AP) is an infection that causes inflammation and destruction of the periradicular tissues. It happens as a result of a series of assaults on the tooth pulp, such as infection, physical and iatrogenic trauma, endodontic therapy, and the destructive effects of root canal filling materials [7]. Then, the host mounts a slew of defenses, including various cell types, intercellular messengers, antibodies, and effector chemicals. Microbial factors and host defense forces interact with, battle with, and destroy much of the periapical tissue, resulting in the production of several types of AP lesions, most often reactive granulomas and cysts, with simultaneous bone resorption around the roots of impacted teeth.

Periodontitis or dental trauma can result in periodontal tissue destruction. It is the destruction of the tooth-supporting structures especially the PDL, and alveolar bone leading to the recession of the marginal gingiva, root exposure, tooth mobility and drifting, and, eventually, tooth loss. They are the results of chronic periodontitis with host defense response, tissue inflammation, and bone destruction in response to bacterial aggression [8]. Especially, the receptor activator of nuclear factor – (KB) ligand (RANKL) is a member of the TNF cytokine family encoded by the gene TNFSF11. It expresses in a membrane-bound protein or secreted forms and plays an important role in bone resorption including periodontal bone destruction via cellular and immune responses under the term the cross-talk between bone biology and immunology - osteoimmunology [9, 10].

3. Cellular responses in periodontal tissue destruction

3.1 Immune cell responses

The first physical barrier that is against infection from bacterial invasion is the periodontal epithelium. The epithelial barriers prevent pathogenic invasion and protect the periodontal tissues. The cells are involved in an active role in the innate host defense as well as further acquired immune responses. When the pathogens overcome the fence, they cause inflammation and destruction of the connective tissue, with subsequent bone loss and tooth loss. In periodontal tissues, cytokines are produced by fibroblasts, endothelial cells, macrophages, osteoclasts, epithelial cells, and leukocytes. By those mediators, osteoclasts will be differentiated and accumulated to the injury (**Figure 2**) [12].

The cells of the adaptive immune system are special types of leukocytes, called lymphocytes. They produce a number of mediators of signaling to induce osteoclastogenesis, such as IL-1, -6, and -17; RANKL; and TNF-α. The differentiation of osteoclast is mainly regulated by RANKL and macrophage-colony stimulating factor (M-CSF). Both of these factors are secreted by immune cells and osteoblasts, odontoblasts, osteoclasts, and other cells in the PDL during alveolar bone resorption [13]. On the other hand, osteoprotegerin (OPG) is a member of the TNF receptor superfamily that prevents osteoclast differentiation, as well as its resorptive function, and stimulates osteoclast apoptosis. It is found in PDL cells and osteoblasts while Receptor activator of nuclear factor κ B (RANK) is detected in osteoclasts and osteoclast precursors. In normal bone remodeling and a variety of pathologic circumstances, RANKL/RANK signaling directs the generation of multinucleated osteoclasts from their progenitors, as well as their activation and survival. By attaching to RANKL and inhibiting it from connecting to its receptor, RANK, OPG protects the skeleton from excessive bone resorption. As a result, the RANKL/OPG ratio is a key predictor of bone mass and skeletal integrity [14].

Early, Baker et al. [15] found that following *Porphyromonas gingivalis* infection in periodontal disease, CD4+ T cells and their proinflammatory cytokines are important effectors of bone destruction as an adaptive immune response [15]. Directly, CD4+ T cells are the primary cells responsible for the increased levels of RANKL in chronic periodontitis patients contributing to the molecular local imbalance that

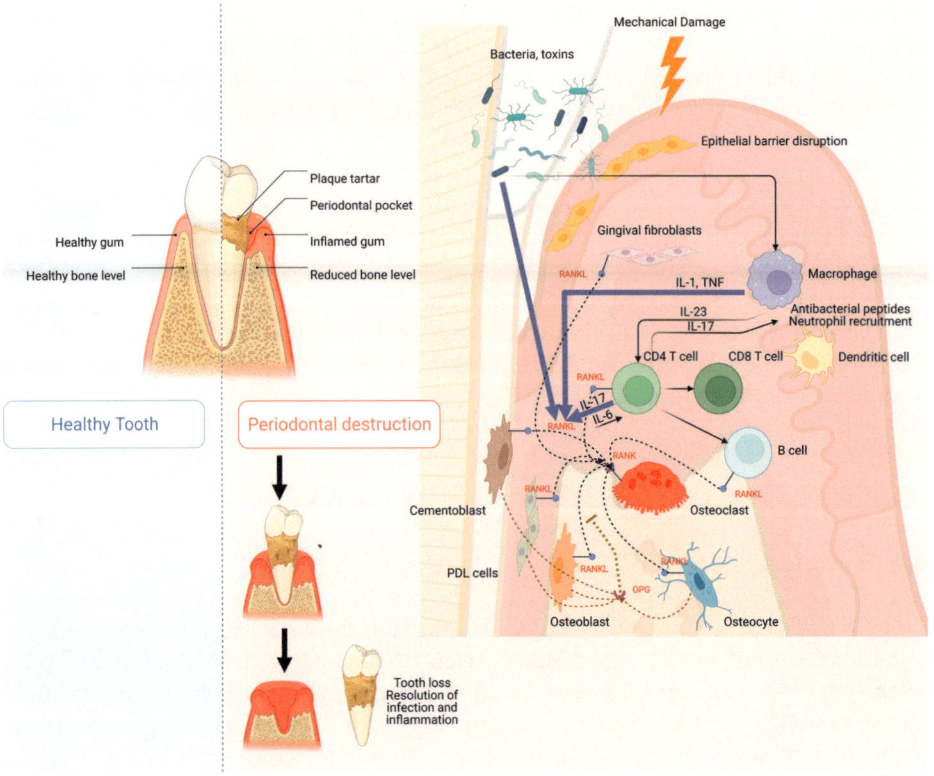

Figure 2.
The mechanisms involved in periodontal tissue destruction. The breakdown of the epithelial barriers by infection or mechanical damage allows bacteria and their toxins to enter and stimulates the immune response. The OPG/RANKL/RANK system plays a central role in regulating bone destruction in periodontal tissue. RANKL binds to the RANK receptor on osteoclast precursor to activate osteoclast while OPG neutralizes this interaction to inhibit osteoclastogenesis. RANKL was main produced by periodontal stromal cells, such as gingival fibroblasts, PDL cells, cementoblasts, osteoblasts, and especially osteocytes as well as immune cells, such as T cells and B cells. T cells communicate with other cells, such as stromal cells, macrophages, and dendritic cells via IL-17, IL-6, and IL-23 to regulate RANKL/OPG signaling resulting in bone destruction and tooth loss and resolution of infection and inflammation [9, 11]. Created with BioRender.com.

results in periodontitis-induced alveolar bone resorption [16]. Besides the ability to support osteoclastogenesis directly, T lymphocytes secrete IL-1, IL-6, and IL-17 which can stimulate RANKL expression. The cells also inhibit osteoclast formation by a number of inhibitory molecules such as IL-4, -10, and -13 ... and IFN-γ [17]. Horwood 2001 [18] inhibited osteoclast formation in cocultures of rat and human cells treated with M-CSF and RANKL by IL-12 and IL-18. When they were administered at synergistically low doses both GM-CSF and IFN-γ were secreted. T helper cells also play role in determining the effect of the T lymphocytes' immune responses against periodontal diseases. Bainbridge et al. 2010 [19] tested the capacity of some *P. gingivalis* strains to induce gingival inflammation, immune responses, and alveolar bone resorption of periodontal disease. They found that these certain strains can induce significant systemic levels of IgG and isotypes IgG1, IgG2a, and IgG2b, indicating the involvement of both two types of T helper cell responses to infection.

In the bone resorption lesion of periodontal disease, regulatory T cell (Treg, FoxP3 + CD25+) was diminished and associated with the increased RANKL+ T cells [20].

Using animal models, Treg recruiting in periodontal tissue can inhibit periodontitis, however, Treg's function might be suppressed [21]. Intriguingly, under inflammatory conditions, several Tregs can convert into Th17 cells called exFoxp3Th17 cells, which induce strongly osteoclastogenesis and bone destruction via IL-17 production [22]. These cells are also found in periodontal lesions in response to the oral commensal bacteria and play a central role in periodontal inflammation [23].

It was known that B cells and plasma cells are also able to produce RANKL to induce osteoclastogenesis [24, 25]. However, there was little evidence of the role of B cells in osteoclastogenesis. In the absence of T lymphocytes, *Actinobacillus actinomycetemcomitans*-responsive B lymphocytes can lead to accelerate periodontal bone resorption via the up-regulation of RANKL [26, 27]. In brief, bacterial antigen-specific T and B lymphocytes play a key role in RANKL- mediated bone loss in periodontal tissue destruction [24].

3.2 Non-immune cell responses

Regarding these oral pathogens, in PDL cells, *P. gingivalis* and/or nicotine activation increased reactive oxygen species (ROS) and superoxide production indicating oxidative stress [28]. It was confirmed clinically in the saliva of patients with chronic periodontitis [29, 30]. In gingival fibroblasts, high concentrations of saline (NaCl) inhibited cell migration but not proliferation [31]. These findings highlighted the susceptibility of these periodontal fibroblasts under oral stimulating factors. Injury to the periapical tissue can damage periodontal cells (gingival fibroblasts, PDL cells, cementoblasts), resulting in the production of cementoclasts/osteoclasts locally. *P. gingivalis* upregulated the RANKL expression in gingival fibroblasts and PDL cells, denoting enhanced osteoclastogenesis [32].

We previously separated cementoblasts from human third molars and co-cultivating them with mononuclear blood cells. Both osteoclast development and resorptive activity were studied in the absence and presence of IL-1. Cementoblasts could initiate osteoclastogenesis via RANKL production, which is heavily influenced by IL-1β explaining why osteoclasts can arise around the root of teeth [33]. RANKL was also produced primarily by osteocytes during the alveolar bone remodeling of the orthodontic tooth movement process. Using a newly developed approach for isolating periodontal tissue component cells from the alveolar bone, Shoji-Matsunaga et al. discovered that osteocytes expressed far more RANKL than other periodontal tissue cells [34]. The decrease of orthodontic tooth movement in mice particularly missing RANKL in osteocytes demonstrated the crucial function of osteocyte-derived RANKL. The study highlighted the critical involvement of osteocyte-derived RANKL in alveolar bone remodeling, laying the groundwork for orthodontic force-mediated bone resorption.

3.3 Pro-inflammatory molecule responses

Pro-inflammatory molecules including chemokines, interleukins, and TNF (Tumor Necrosis Factors) were secreted by immune and stromal cells during the inflammation and bone resorption of periodontal tissue destruction. Chemokines are chemotactic cytokines that stimulate the recruitment of inflammatory cells. Chemokines have a role in osteoclastogenesis by inducing the differentiation of osteoclasts, they also affect osteoclast functions/properties [35]. In this way, chemokines can affect periodontal bone loss by recruiting neutrophils to fight against bacteria. Yu et al. [36] use *P. gingivalis* in CXCR2-deficient mice, a type of chemokine receptor. The result showed that knockout mice were highly susceptible to alveolar bone loss. These mice also suggested a role for chemokines in maintaining normal bone homeostasis.

Interleukins are a group of cytokines that are expressed by leukocytes and function in the immune system. Many studies in human and animal patterns have indicated the mediating bone loss stimulated by periodontal pathogens. Delima [17] investigated the role of IL-1 in periodontal disease in monkeys by using an inhibitor. The results indicate that inhibition of IL-1 significantly reduces inflammation, connective tissue attachment loss, and bone resorption. Especially, the transgenic mice that overexpress a form of IL-1α in the oral mucosal epithelium develop a syndrome that possesses all of the major features of periodontal disease, including epithelial proliferation and apical migration, loss of attachment, and destruction of cementum and alveolar bone [37]. Using antibiotics did not reduce the disease, giving the role of IL-1 in mediating in promoting the destruction of the periodontium. However, other types of IL seem to reduce bone loss and symptoms of disease in the periodontium. For example, according to Shaker 2012 [38], the IL-11 concentration was significantly higher in control and chronic periodontitis groups in comparison to aggressive periodontitis groups.

Curiously, studies reported the opposing roles of IL-17 in periodontal bone resorption, especially with rheumatoid arthritis (RA) condition. Th17 cells produce mainly IL-17 leading to bone destruction in RA by mediating the osteoclastogenesis process [38, 39]. However, inflammatory mediators, including chemokines, cytokines, prostaglandin E2, and nitric oxide that IL-17 recruited in RA conditions have antibacterial properties that lead to bone protection in the context of periodontal infection. Yu et al. [36] examined IL-17's role in inflammatory bone loss induced by *P. gingivalis* in IL-17–deficient mice in an autoimmune arthritis model. These animals had increased periodontal bone degradation, indicating that IL-17 has a bone-protective effect.

TNF refers to a group of cytokines that can cause cell death. In this family, TNF-α has various functions, such as cytolysis of some specific cells, cachexia, pyrogen, cell proliferation, and differentiation in some cases. It seems to be that reducing the level of TNF-α in the body leads to reduce bone loss, however, it will increase the number of bacteria in the lesion since the lessen immune response. Garlet et al. [40] examined how TNF-α modulates the periodontal disease by *A. actinomycetemcomitans* in TNF-α receptor-deficient mice. These mice had less severe periodontitis with less alveolar bone loss and inflammatory reaction. However, the higher level of bacteria compares with the wild-type group.

4. Relation in dental practice

Implants, orthodontics, and other areas of maxillofacial dentistry are more or less based on the predictable repair and regeneration of the bone and supporting tissues around the teeth. In the field of implantology, the process of bone repair and regeneration (osteogenesis) plays an important role in determining the success of treatment. Bone integration includes the initial stages of tissue response, peri-implant osteogenesis, and peri-implant bone remodeling, resulting in new bone formation on the implant surface. Composition, implant design, and surface treatment affect bone integration. Other factors include systemic condition, surgical technique, adequate healing time, and load-bearing properties. In dental implants, bone and implant integrate directly (**Figure 3**). There are no PDL and Sharpey's fibers that help to absorb force and micro trauma. Instead, osteoblasts are attached to the mineralized collagen framework, forming a dense, mineralized area directly on the implant surface. The distance from the bone to the implant surface takes place in a continuous process of bone regeneration in response to stress and mechanical force over time. The cavity containing osteoclasts, osteoblasts, mesenchymal cells, and blood vessels is always present adjacent to the implant surface [41, 42]. Excessive micro-motion in healing leads to tension and torsion forces, stimulating the formation of a fibrin membrane around the implant, and displacing the bone-implant interface. This phenomenon loosens the implant, inhibiting bone integration.

Using the bone repair and regeneration processes to accelerate tooth movement in orthodontics can significantly reduce treatment time and harmful effects. The ability to move teeth is mainly determined by the regeneration of periodontal tissue, under the regulation of molecular mechanisms by the response of cells in the alveolar bone and PDL. Fluid shear stress that PDL cells are constantly subjected to, is a form of mechanical loading on the cell level. Under compression, the fluids are forced through the voids and are relocated either to adjacent zones of the PDL or driven into the neighboring alveolar bone. This fluid movement creates the type of mechanical

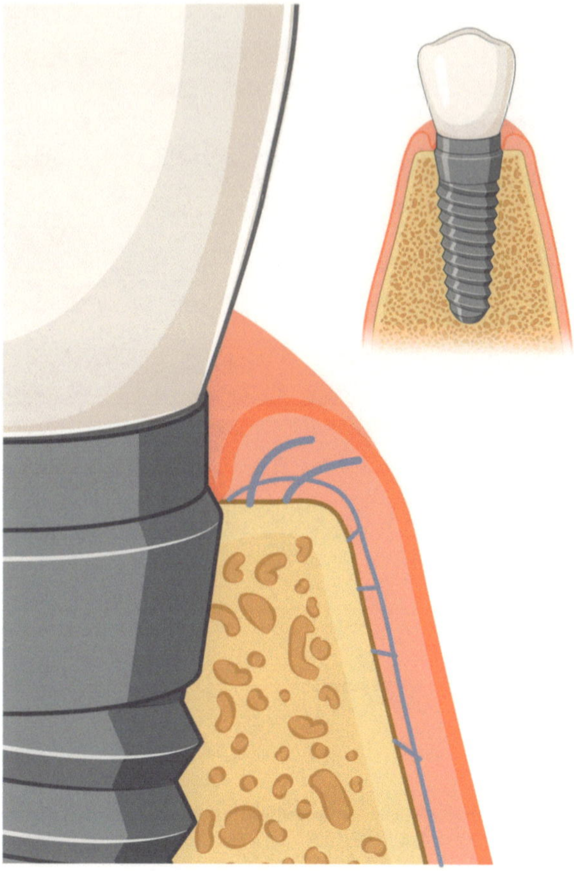

Figure 3.
*The anchor of a dental implant in the alveolar bone directly by the osteointegration without the PDL and Sharpey's fibers in comparison to the real teeth (**Figure 1**). Note that there was also no connective tissue connection between the implant and the gingiva. Created with BioRender.com.*

loading known as fluid shear stress [43]. This force appears during the mastication, speech, and orthodontic procedure. By their arrangement and structure, fibers of PDL can absorb forces that are harmful to teeth and surrounding apparatus. However, excessing the endured limitation of PDL (by duration and/or magnitude), PDL can respond to the compression by stimulating many compartments. By using mechanical stress (light orthodontic application) to activate the fluid shear stress response in PDL cells, Yarmolyuk 2012 [44] showed that it could alleviate the compromised periodontal status via down-regulation of TLR4.

Similar to the inflammation response triggered by bacteria, mechanical forces also cause increased cytokine secretion by PDL cells. By using an orthodontic model which can mimic real situations, many studies have proven that IL-1β, IL-6, and TNF-α have been revealed in the compression side of teeth [45]. In the results of this elevation, the OPG/RANKL/RANK system will function leading to bone remodeling. Depending on the kind of force and its magnitude, the bone will be resorbed or formed prominently (**Figure 4**).

Interestingly, Diercke et al. [46] indicated that static compressive forces significantly induced the expression of ephrin-A2, while the expression of ephrin -B2 was significantly down-regulated in PDL. Although these coupling factors (Ephrin and eph receptor) have been defined as osteoclast-derived molecules that induce

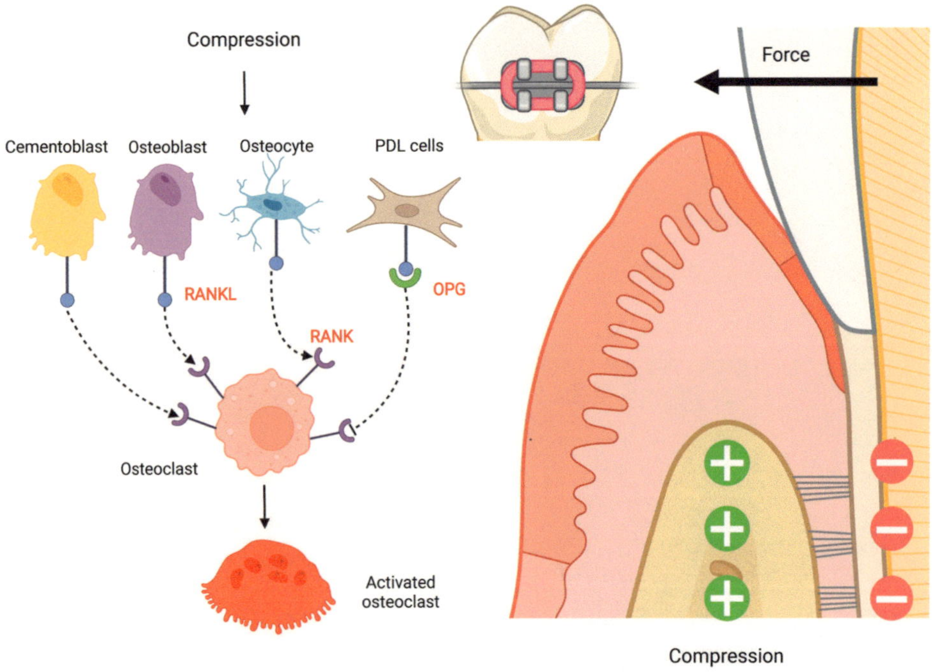

Figure 4.
Orthodontics force induces periodontal and bone tissue remodeling. Mechanical stress applied to a tooth can destruct periodontal and bone tissue through the RANKL/RANK/OPG system. At the site of compression, periodontal tissue cells such as PDL cells, cementoblasts, osteoblasts, and osteocytes of alveolar bone can produce RANKL to active osteoclast via RANK leading to bone resorption. On the opposite side of the tooth where OPG will be produced increasingly by stromal cells to inhibit osteoclastogenesis leading to more bone formation. The application of too strong orthodontics force will enhance uncontrolled osteoclastogenesis/cementoclastogenesis leading to tooth's root resorption (external resorption) and periodontal tissue destruction permanently. Created with BioRender.com.

osteoblastic bone formation. The more ephrin-A2, the more osteoclast, while reducing ephrin-B2 will reduce osteoblast formation [47].

Low-level lasers can also accelerate tooth migration, according to human and animal studies [48–52]. However, some studies suggest that low-level lasers do not accelerate tooth migration but also slow it down [53]. This difference may be explained by different treatment regimens including laser wavelength, radiation dose, location, and frequency. Several studies have reported that low-level lasers stimulate bone regeneration by increasing the number and function of osteoblasts and osteoclasts as well as markers, such as matrix metalloproteinase-9, cathepsin K, integrin [50], and the RANK/RANKL/OPG system [51, 54] at periodontal tissue. More research is needed to find the most effective regimen to extend its effectiveness.

5. Conclusions

The imbalance between bone resorption and formation leads to the loss of bone and PDL. This process is regulated by inflammatory infiltration followed by a dozen of factors, such as bacterial products, cytokines, chemokines, and complements from surrounding cells and blood vessels. Using our knowledge of periodontal tissue destruction, bone repair, and regeneration mechanisms, and the factors that influence them help us to better understand the molecular mechanisms, explain phenomena and applications, and develop approaches to new treatments, thereby helping to achieve optimal treatment results, and minimizing complications for patients.

Acknowledgements

The author thanks the Faculty of Odonto-Stomatology, University of Medicine and Pharmacy at Ho Chi Minh City, Vietnam for supporting this chapter.

Conflict of interest

The author declares that there is no conflict of interest regarding the publication of this chapter.

Author details

Nam Cong-Nhat Huynh
Faculty of Odonto-Stomatology, Laboratory of Prosthodontics, Laboratory of Oral-Maxillofacial Biology, University of Medicine and Pharmacy at Ho Chi Minh City, Ho Chi Minh City, Vietnam

*Address all correspondence to: namhuynh@ump.edu.vn; huynhcongnhatnam@gmail.com

References

[1] Melcher AH. On the repair potential of periodontal tissues. Journal of Periodontology. 1976;**47**(5):256-260

[2] Rathee M, Jain P. Embryology, Teeth. Treasure Island (FL): StatPearls; 2022

[3] Seo BM, Song IS, Um S, Lee J-H. Chapter 22 - Periodontal ligament stem cells. In: Vishwakarma A, Sharpe P, Shi S, Ramalingam M, editors. Stem Cell Biology and Tissue Engineering in Dental Sciences. Boston: Academic Press; 2015. pp. 291-296

[4] Cho MI, Garant PR. Development and general structure of the periodontium. Periodontology 2000. 2000;**2000**(24):9-27

[5] Nguyen TT, Ho TH, Huynh CN, Dien HAV, Vo LT. Hyaluronic acid 0.2% application enhanced periodontitis treatment in non-surgical phase. Journal of Stomatology. 2021;**74**(2):76-83

[6] Kinane DF, Stathopoulou PG, Papapanou PN. Periodontal diseases. Nature Reviews Disease Primers. 2017;**3**:17038

[7] Graunaite I, Lodiene G, Maciulskiene V. Pathogenesis of apical periodontitis: A literature review. Journal of Oral & Maxillofacial Research. 2012;**2**(4):e1

[8] Bascones A, Noronha S, Gomez M, Mota P, Gonzalez Moles MA, Villarroel DM. Tissue destruction in periodontitis: Bacteria or cytokines fault? Quintessence International. 2005;**36**(4):299-306

[9] Tsukasaki M. RANKL and osteoimmunology in periodontitis. Journal of Bone and Mineral Metabolism. 2021;**39**(1):82-90

[10] Chen B, Wu W, Sun W, Zhang Q, Yan F, Xiao Y. RANKL expression in periodontal disease: Where does RANKL come from? BioMed Research International. 2014;**2014**:731039

[11] Tsukasaki M, Takayanagi H. Osteoimmunology: Evolving concepts in bone-immune interactions in health and disease. Nature Reviews. Immunology. 2019;**19**(10):626-642

[12] Mariano FS, de Cássia Orlandi Sardi J, Duque C, Höfling JF, Gonçalves RB. The role of immune system in the development of periodontal disease: A brief review. Revista Odonto Ciência. 2010;**25**(3):300-305

[13] Tyrovola JB, Spyropoulos MN, Makou M, Perrea D. Root resorption and the OPG/RANKL/RANK system: A mini review. Journal of Oral Science. 2008;**50**(4):367-376

[14] Boyce BF, Xing L. Biology of RANK, RANKL, and osteoprotegerin. Arthritis Research & Therapy. 2007;**9**(Suppl. 1):S1

[15] Baker PJ, Dixon M, Evans RT, Dufour L, Johnson E, Roopenian DC. CD4(+) T cells and the proinflammatory cytokines gamma interferon and interleukin-6 contribute to alveolar bone loss in mice. Infection and Immunity. 1999;**67**(6):2804-2809

[16] Vernal R, Dutzan N, Hernandez M, Chandia S, Puente J, Leon R, et al. High expression levels of receptor activator of nuclear factor-kappa B ligand associated with human chronic periodontitis are mainly secreted by CD4+ T lymphocytes. Journal of Periodontology. 2006;**77**(10):1772-1780

[17] Delima AJ, Karatzas S, Amar S, Graves DT. Inflammation and tissue

loss caused by periodontal pathogens is reduced by interleukin-1 antagonists. The Journal of Infectious Diseases. 2002;**186**(4):511-516

[18] Horwood NJ, Elliott J, Martin TJ, Gillespie MT. IL-12 alone and in synergy with IL-18 inhibits osteoclast formation in vitro. Journal of Immunology. 2001;**166**(8):4915-4921

[19] Bainbridge B, Verma RK, Eastman C, Yehia B, Rivera M, Moffatt C, et al. Role of Porphyromonas gingivalis phosphoserine phosphatase enzyme SerB in inflammation, immune response, and induction of alveolar bone resorption in rats. Infection and Immunity. 2010;**78**(11):4560-4569

[20] Ernst CW, Lee JE, Nakanishi T, Karimbux NY, Rezende TM, Stashenko P, et al. Diminished forkhead box P3/CD25 double-positive T regulatory cells are associated with the increased nuclear factor-kappaB ligand (RANKL+) T cells in bone resorption lesion of periodontal disease. Clinical and Experimental Immunology. 2007;**148**(2):271-280

[21] Glowacki AJ, Yoshizawa S, Jhunjhunwala S, Vieira AE, Garlet GP, Sfeir C, et al. Prevention of inflammation-mediated bone loss in murine and canine periodontal disease via recruitment of regulatory lymphocytes. Proceedings of the National Academy of Sciences of the United States of America. 2013;**110**(46):18525-18530

[22] Komatsu N, Okamoto K, Sawa S, Nakashima T, Oh-hora M, Kodama T, et al. Pathogenic conversion of Foxp3+ T cells into TH17 cells in autoimmune arthritis. Nature Medicine. 2014;**20**(1):62-68

[23] Tsukasaki M, Komatsu N, Nagashima K, Nitta T, Pluemsakunthai W, Shukunami C, et al. Host defense against oral microbiota by bone-damaging T cells. Nature Communications. 2018;**9**(1):701

[24] Kajiya M, Giro G, Taubman MA, Han X, Mayer MP, Kawai T. Role of periodontal pathogenic bacteria in RANKL-mediated bone destruction in periodontal disease. Journal of Oral Microbiology. 2010;**2**

[25] Komatsu N, Win S, Yan M, Huynh NC, Sawa S, Tsukasaki M, et al. Plasma cells promote osteoclastogenesis and periarticular bone loss in autoimmune arthritis. The Journal of Clinical Investigation. 2021;**131**(6)

[26] Han X, Kawai T, Eastcott JW, Taubman MA. Bacterial-responsive B lymphocytes induce periodontal bone resorption. Journal of Immunology. 2006;**176**(1):625-631

[27] Han X, Lin X, Seliger AR, Eastcott J, Kawai T, Taubman MA. Expression of receptor activator of nuclear factor-kappaB ligand by B cells in response to oral bacteria. Oral Microbiology and Immunology. 2009;**24**(3):190-196

[28] Nguyen TT, Huynh NN, Seubbuk S, Nilmoje T, Wanasuntronwong A, Surarit R. Oxidative stress induced by Porphyromonas gingivalis lysate and nicotine in human periodontal ligament fibroblasts. Odontology. 2019;**107**(2):133-141

[29] Nguyen TT, Vo DA, Thai TT, Vo TL, Huynh NC. Total oxidant status and total antioxidant capacity in the saliva of patients with chronic periodontitis. Medical and Pharmaceutical Researches. 2020;**4**(4):21-26

[30] Zhang T, Andrukhov O, Haririan H, Muller-Kern M, Liu S, Liu Z, et al. Total antioxidant capacity and total oxidant

status in saliva of periodontitis patients in relation to bacterial load. Frontiers in Cellular and Infection Microbiology. 2015;**5**:97

[31] Huynh NC, Everts V, Leethanakul C, Pavasant P, Ampornaramveth RS. Rinsing with saline promotes human gingival fibroblast wound healing in vitro. PLoS One. 2016;**11**(7):e0159843

[32] Belibasakis GN, Bostanci N, Hashim A, Johansson A, Aduse-Opoku J, Curtis MA, et al. Regulation of RANKL and OPG gene expression in human gingival fibroblasts and periodontal ligament cells by Porphyromonas gingivalis: A putative role of the Arg-gingipains. Microbial Pathogenesis. 2007;**43**(1):46-53

[33] Huynh NC, Everts V, Pavasant P, Ampornaramveth RS. Interleukin-1beta induces human cementoblasts to support osteoclastogenesis. International Journal of Oral Science. 2017;**9**(12):e5

[34] Shoji-Matsunaga A, Ono T, Hayashi M, Takayanagi H, Moriyama K, Nakashima T. Osteocyte regulation of orthodontic force-mediated tooth movement via RANKL expression. Scientific Reports. 2017;**7**(1):8753

[35] Silva TA, Garlet GP, Fukada SY, Silva JS, Cunha FQ. Chemokines in oral inflammatory diseases: Apical periodontitis and periodontal disease. Journal of Dental Research. 2007;**86**(4):306-319

[36] Yu JJ, Ruddy MJ, Wong GC, Sfintescu C, Baker PJ, Smith JB, et al. An essential role for IL-17 in preventing pathogen-initiated bone destruction: Recruitment of neutrophils to inflamed bone requires IL-17 receptor-dependent signals. Blood. 2007;**109**(9):3794-3802

[37] Dayan S, Stashenko P, Niederman R, Kupper TS. Oral epithelial overexpression of IL-1alpha causes periodontal disease. Journal of Dental Research. 2004;**83**(10):786-790

[38] Shaker OG, Ghallab NA. IL-17 and IL-11 GCF levels in aggressive and chronic periodontitis patients: Relation to PCR bacterial detection. Mediators of Inflammation. 2012;**2012**:174764

[39] Gaffen SL. Biology of recently discovered cytokines: Interleukin-17--a unique inflammatory cytokine with roles in bone biology and arthritis. Arthritis Research & Therapy. 2004;**6**(6):240-247

[40] Garlet GP, Cardoso CR, Campanelli AP, Ferreira BR, Avila-Campos MJ, Cunha FQ, et al. The dual role of p55 tumour necrosis factor-alpha receptor in Actinobacillus actinomycetemcomitans-induced experimental periodontitis: Host protection and tissue destruction. Clinical and Experimental Immunology. 2007;**147**(1):128-138

[41] Mavrogenis A, Dimitriou R, Parvizi J, Babis GC. Biology of implant osseointegration. Journal of Musculoskeletal & Neuronal Interactions. 2009;**9**(2):61-71

[42] Mulari M, Qu Q, Härkönen P, Väänänen H. Osteoblast-like cells complete osteoclastic bone resorption and form new mineralized bone matrix in vitro. Calcified Tissue International. 2004;**75**(3):253-261

[43] Bergomi M, Cugnoni J, Galli M, Botsis J, Belser UC, Wiskott HW. Hydro-mechanical coupling in the periodontal ligament: A porohyperelastic finite element model. Journal of Biomechanics. 2011;**44**(1):34-38

[44] Yarmolyuk Y. Mechanical Stress Modulates Expression of Toll-Like

Receptors in Human PDL. Milwaukee, Wisconsin: Marquette University; 2012

[45] Diercke K, Kohl A, Lux CJ, Erber R. IL-1beta and compressive forces lead to a significant induction of RANKL-expression in primary human cementoblasts. Journal of Orofacial Orthopedics = Fortschritte der Kieferorthopadie: Organ/Official Journal Deutsche Gesellschaft fur Kieferorthopadie. 2012;**73**(5):397-412

[46] Diercke K, Sen S, Kohl A, Lux CJ, Erber R. Compression-dependent up-regulation of ephrin-A2 in PDL fibroblasts attenuates osteogenesis. Journal of Dental Research. 2011;**90**(9):1108-1115

[47] Matsuo K, Otaki N. Bone cell interactions through Eph/ephrin: Bone modeling, remodeling and associated diseases. Cell Adhesion & Migration. 2012;**6**(2):148-156

[48] Kawasaki K, Shimizu N. Effects of low-energy laser irradiation on bone remodeling during experimental tooth movement in rats. Lasers in Surgery and Medicine: The Official Journal of the American Society for Laser Medicine and Surgery. 2000;**26**(3):282-291

[49] Sun X, Zhu X, Xu C, Ye N, Zhu H. Effects of low energy laser on tooth movement and remodeling of alveolar bone in rabbits. Hua xi kou qiang yi xue za zhi= Huaxi kouqiang yixue zazhi=. West China Journal of Stomatology. 2001;**19**(5):290-293

[50] Yamaguchi M, Hayashi M, Fujita S, Yoshida T, Utsunomiya T, Yamamoto H, et al. Low-energy laser irradiation facilitates the velocity of tooth movement and the expressions of matrix metalloproteinase-9, cathepsin K, and alpha (v) beta (3) integrin in rats. The European Journal of Orthodontics. 2010;**32**(2):131-139

[51] Fujita S, Yamaguchi M, Utsunomiya T, Yamamoto H, Kasai K. Low-energy laser stimulates tooth movement velocity via expression of RANK and RANKL. Orthodontics & Craniofacial Research. 2008;**11**(3):143-155

[52] Cruz DR, Kohara EK, Ribeiro MS, Wetter NU. Effects of low-intensity laser therapy on the orthodontic movement velocity of human teeth: A preliminary study. Lasers in Surgery and Medicine: The Official Journal of the American Society for Laser Medicine and Surgery. 2004;**35**(2):117-120

[53] Seifi M, Shafeei HA, Daneshdoost S, Mir M. Effects of two types of low-level laser wave lengths (850 and 630 nm) on the orthodontic tooth movements in rabbits. Lasers in Medical Science. 2007;**22**(4):261-264

[54] Zhu X, Chen Y, Sun X. A study on expression of basic fibroblast growth factors in periodontal tissue following orthodontic tooth movement associated with low power laser irradiation. Hua xi kou qiang yi xue za zhi= Huaxi kouqiang yixue zazhi=. West China Journal of Stomatology. 2002;**20**(3):166-168

Chapter 7

Non-Surgical Treatment of Periodontal Diseases: Responsibilities of the Dentist and the Patient in Periodontal Therapy

Luis V. Maita-Véliz and Luis M. Maita-Castañeda

Abstract

Periodontal diseases, throughout history, remain among the most prevalent in humans. Despite the notable scientific advances in the knowledge of its etiology and pathophysiology, its clinical forms, diagnosis and corresponding treatment, the most transcendental stage has yet to be completed: making not only patients in particular, but the entire community aware of the need for surveillance and prevention of periodontal diseases in children, adolescents and adults. Developing a wide-ranging periodic program, with effective and sufficient procedures to anticipate the onset of periodontal diseases, would mean enormous economic savings in the public health budget of the countries. Periodontal diseases can be avoided with simple measures and procedures: correct brushing and good use of dental floss. Both practices would be enough to prevent periodontal diseases in millions of people around the planet. It is a challenge for dental professionals to achieve, through appropriate teaching techniques, that their patients learn these notions and their benefits, thus gradually turning them into essential and daily tasks. The basic objective of promotion and prevention is precisely to ensure that the information produces changes in individual oral hygiene habits.

Keywords: gingivitis, periodontitis, prevention, periodontal hygiene, non-surgical treatment

1. Introduction

Periodontal diseases are one of the most prevalent in humans. In most countries, this index is high and has been maintained for years without major changes.

What agent or phenomenon motivates them? Basically: bacterial plaque or biofilm. Who should control that bacterial plaque? First of all, the affected person. What should you do? Exercise continuous care of your teeth.

It is worth clarifying that there are also adjuvants of a genetic or environmental nature, specific to the patient or their living conditions. These adjuvants modulate the course of periodontal diseases or infections [1, 2].

The basic periodontal therapeutic method continues to be the removal of biofilm from supragingival and/or subgingival spaces or areas, through well-known therapeutic procedures: periodontal hygiene, scaling, and root planning [3].

Non-surgical periodontal treatment is "the cornerstone of periodontal therapy or the gold standard" and is the essential procedure to combat periodontal infections [3].

Phase I is a therapy related to the cause, and therefore, the entire chronological sequence of a periodontal treatment should be initiated [4]. In many cases, only the complete fulfillment of Phase 1 is sufficient to recover periodontal health, with which it makes any other procedure in this regard dispensable.

This phase becomes a critical and fundamental part of periodontal treatment, in general. First of all, it prepares the conditions for the dentist to control the bacterial plaque or biofilm. For this, it instills and strengthens the patient the importance and the way to eliminate the biofilm. Otherwise, you will continue to lose periodontal tissues, even after surgical procedures have been carried out to heal them.

Secondly, it offers the professional the opportunity to observe and evaluate the reaction or response of the periodontal tissues to the phase, with which he can recommend reinforcements, such as careful care at home, which allows him/her to know the periodontal hygiene habits of the patient, and discuss them with him.

2. Bacterial plaque control

It is essential for all types of therapy. This control must be assumed by the patient with full knowledge of what he/she must do about it and awareness of its importance [5].

Oral hygiene methods at home are fundamentally oriented toward the elimination of supragingival plaque and the maintenance of good oral health [6].

The lasting success of effective clinical treatment depends mainly on the collaboration of the patient, who is often unaware of this responsibility [7].

We must carefully and affectionately explain to the patient the nature of the biofilm and the reasons why it needs to be removed for periodontal therapy to be successful “Learning is experience, everything else is information” Einstein.

The patient must be guided in the selection of the most suitable instruments for their individual needs and instructed on the correct way to perform oral hygiene.

The time dedicated to the teaching of these actions and to the conviction of assuming the changes by the patient will depend on the individual needs of the same. It is not an easy task, the patient is not aware of the importance of having good periodontal health and updating their information on hygiene habits. In general, he/she does not know beyond what he learned as a child [8].

Each patient deserves personalized guidance. It is essential to always schedule enough time to explain the techniques and verify the learning of it. The use of audiovisual teaching materials is also recommended to better integrate and/or clarify home oral hygiene methods. It is convenient to suggest:

- A method of brushing (with a manual or electric brush).

- A cleaning instrument for the interproximal spaces (preferably an interdental brush and/or dental floss, depending on the accessibility of said spaces).

- The use of gauze impregnated with medication, especially for hygiene outside the home [9].

If the patient wishes to use an electric toothbrush, he should be warned about the possible risk of causing non-carious cervical lesions, such as dental abrasions or cervical dentin hypersensitivity.

We must make the patient understand that his/her persevering collaboration will determine the desired result. Letting them know the etiology of the disease will facilitate the teaching of a correct periodontal hygiene technique. This means emphasizing the location or placement of the brush bristles in the gingival sulcus, as indicated by the Bass Technique.

The use of dental floss has an equal or greater role than hygiene with a brush alone. The proximal areas are crucial because periodontal disease begins precisely in these areas, because the junctional epithelium of these interproximal spaces has few layers of epithelial cells, which facilitate their conversion into vulnerable areas for the colonization of periodontal pathogens and the consequent deterioration of periodontal health; in addition, this junctional epithelium is not keratinized.

The classic study by Löe et al., in 1965, demonstrated the close relationship between the accumulation of microbial plaque and the development of gingivitis in humans. The study consisted of absolutely suppressing the means of oral hygiene in a group of volunteers. All the people in the research developed gingivitis in a range of 7–21 days. The predominant composition of the bacterial flora was gram. After 7 days of brushing again, good recovery of gingival health was achieved [10].

The careful and correct control of the supragingival biofilm modifies and affects the development and composition of the subgingival biofilm. This allows for a stable microflora and reduces stone formation [11].

Constant control of biofilm at home, added to visits to the dentist for periodontal prophylaxis and calculus removal, will reduce the amount of supragingival biofilm, decrease the total number of microorganisms sheltered in moderate periodontal pockets and furcation areas, and will finally restrict the abundance of periodontal pathogens [12, 13]. The increase in biofilm or biofilms occurs hour after hour and must be completely removed within 48 hours at most from all places with poor periodontal health to prevent inflammation [14]. The American Dental Association (ADA) recommends brushing teeth twice a day and use dental floss for interproximal cleaning once a day; in this way, we will achieve an effective removal of biofilm and prevent gingivitis [15].

A single brushing removes only part of the dental plaque. Doing it twice ensures better results. Bear in mind that periodontal disease begins and is located in the interproximal spaces, places where precisely a single brushing does not completely exclude bacterial plaque [16].

Another risk factor is that periodontal patients are easily susceptible to periodontal disease, a consequence of complex defects in the gingival architecture, caused by the same periodontal disease that afflicts them and the extensively exposed root surfaces. All this hinders correct periodontal hygiene [17].

The antibacterial agent that has shown the most effective is chlorhexidine. Various investigations have provided evidence that it almost completely inhibits the development of biofilm, calculus, and gingivitis. The most commonly used concentration is 0.12% [18]. Chlorhexidine has some reversible side effects, including slightly darkening resin restorations, tooth surfaces, and the tongue. Chlorhexidine is commonly found as a non-alcoholic preparation. In any form of presentation, it is effective for biofilm control [19].

Likewise, there are natural products that are being investigated and used as adjuvant agents in the control and treatment of periodontal disease [20, 21].

3. Toothbrush

It is an implement that has two parts: a handle and a head. The head has bristles (soft or hard) whose function is to remove, through specific movements, food, and drink residues that adhere to the dental surfaces or are lodged in the adjoining interstices. Toothbrushes come with a wide variety of bristles in terms of size, design, length, hardness, and arrangement (**Figure 1**).

There is no ideal brushing technique for all patients [6].

Patients can use a brushing technique that effectively removes microbial plaque while avoiding trauma to soft tissue. It can be concluded by saying that efficiency is more important than technique [22].

The investigations, regarding the advantages of each one of the brushes, do not determine exactly if there is any superiority in cases of gingivitis or gingival bleeding. A comparative study of four different toothbrushes, in their action of removing biofilm with brushing, showed that the four chosen brushes equally removed biofilm and that a certain configuration was not more effective than another [5] (**Figures 2–4**).

After a systematic review of several studies on toothbrushes, it was concluded that there is no superior or better design between one or the other [24].

The effectiveness and the potential for injury offered by the different types of brushes depend to a large extent, and especially on the technique of use and manual skill.

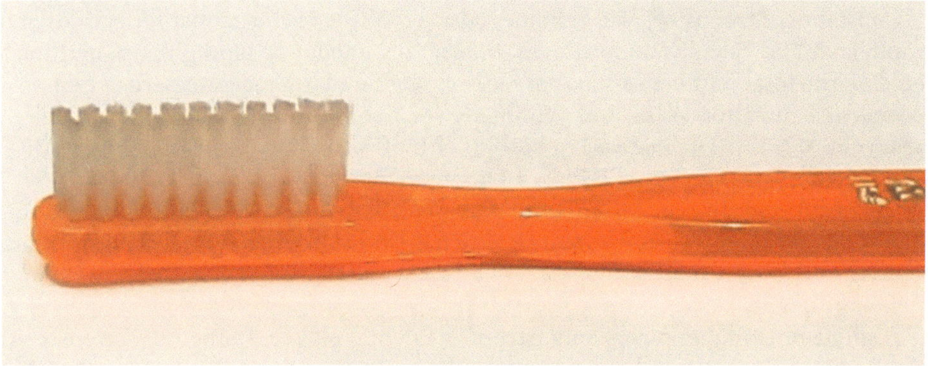

Figure 1.
Straight-handle toothbrush with a head that houses the spaced tufts. The bristles are soft. The edge, at its end, is rounded.

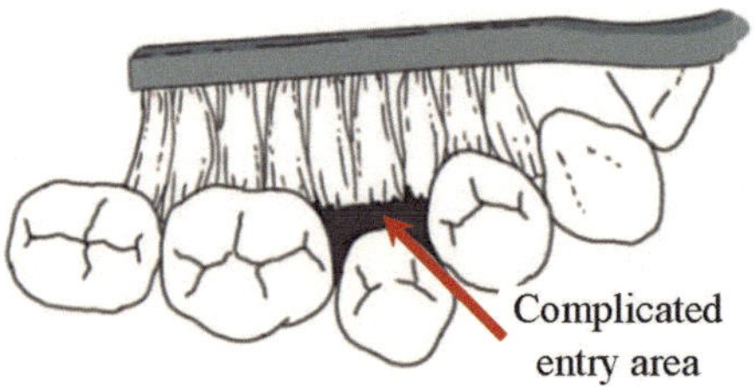

Figure 2.
Difficult access area and, therefore, difficult to clean, if a toothbrush with an excessive number of bristles is used. Adapted from MacPhee T., Cowley G [23].

DOI: http://dx.doi.org/10.5772/intechopen.107332

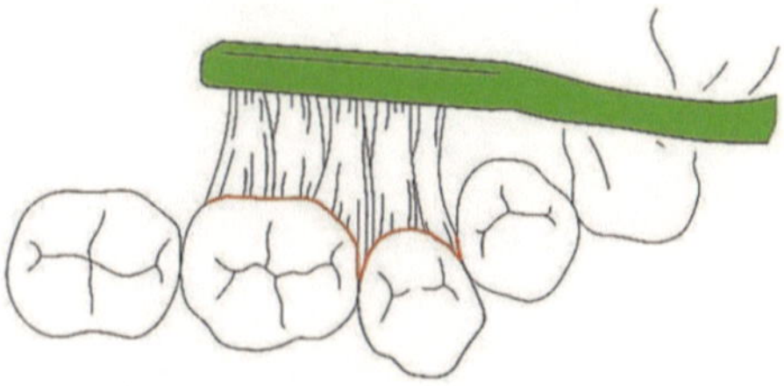

Figure 3.
Toothbrush with a sufficient number of bristles for brushing in complicated areas. Adapted from MacPhee T., Cowley G [23].

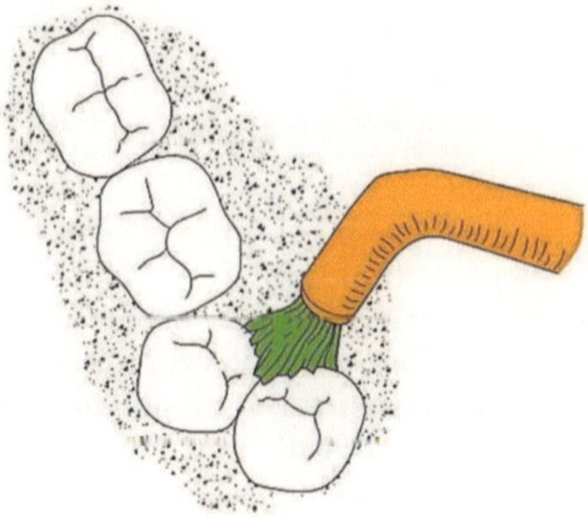

Figure 4.
A plume-type brush can also be used. Adapted from MacPhee T., Cowley G [23].

When used incorrectly, the toothbrush can cause injuries or alterations, both on the dental surface and in the gingival tissues (**Figures 5** and **6**).

The alterations, such as abrasion (non-carious cervical lesions), are related to various dental factors involved in tooth brushing: use of brushes with hard bristles,

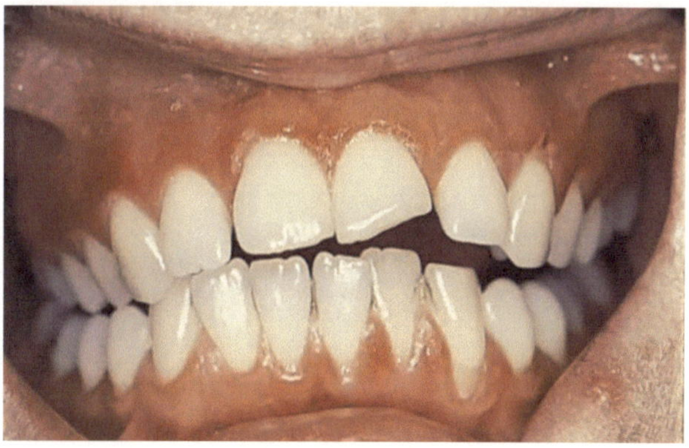

Figure 5.
The patient has brushed to the extreme by applying excessive force. At the gingival margin of maxillary central incisors 1.1 and 2.1, erosive traumatic lesions are observed.

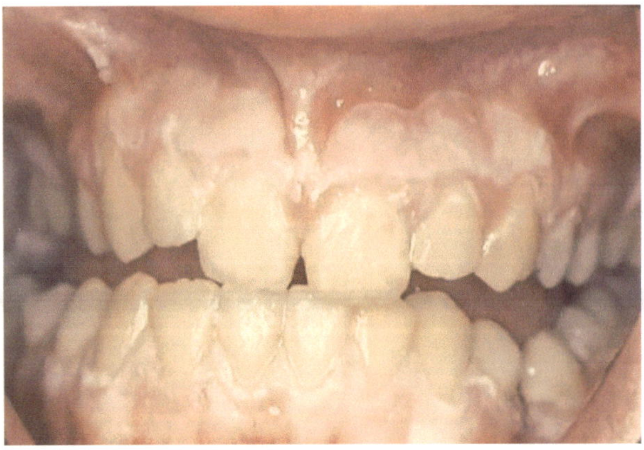

Figure 6.
The patient has not brushed for several days. In both jaws, a whitish layer is noted on the marginal and attached gingiva. It is the accumulation of keratin. When you rub it, it comes off easily. The mucosal surface will not show any alteration and all features are normal.

horizontal brushing applying excessive force, use of toothpaste with highly abrasive substances, poor dental position, and others. Any of these factors can induce the appearance of abrasive cervical lesions and gingival recessions [25].

With some frequency, traumatic injuries to soft and hard tissues are observed, due to the use of inappropriate toothbrushes with hard, uneven, or very worn bristles, and also due to inadequate or incorrect brushing techniques [26] (**Figure** 7).

Pointing out, we will say: bristles with rounded ends cause less damage to gingival tissues than flat-cut bristles with sharp ends [27, 28].

Soft-bristled toothbrushes, described by Bass more than 70 years ago, have gained wide acceptance and continue to be used by the professional dental community [29].

It is very important to consider that in order to recommend a toothbrushing technique, we must clinically assess the keratinization of the gingiva and the periodontal biotype, that is, whether it is a thick or firm biotype [30].

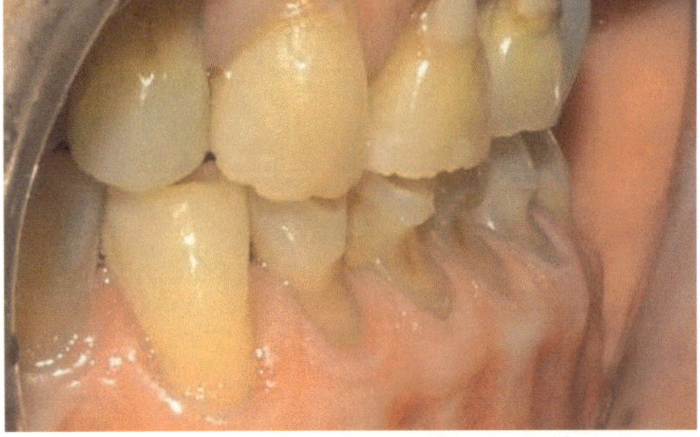

Figure 7.
Patient who, despite being warned of the need to change his/her brushing method, and having been given instructions for an effective brushing technique, did not cooperate in applying it.

There are also electric brushes. They are useful in the following cases: children and adolescents, people with physical or mental disabilities, hospitalized patients including the elderly (elderly) requiring assistant careers, and, in some cases, patients with fixed orthodontia. In the case of children, it is recommended that they first learn to use a regular toothbrush, then an electric toothbrush.

The role of toothpaste is to help clean and polish the surface of the teeth, increasing the effectiveness of brushing. Toothpastes are products that contain various substances, including some abrasives. Abrasives are insoluble inorganic salts. They serve to increase the abrasive action of brushing up to 40 times more and constitute between 20% and 40% of the composition of toothpaste. Oral hygiene procedures that use abrasive toothpaste are the essential cause of hard tissue damage and it is possible that gingival lesions could also be caused by those ingredients [31].

4. Reasons for oral hygiene

Several classic studies show the importance of controlling supragingival bacterial biofilm. Löe et al. unquestionably demonstrated the cause-effect relationship between the accumulation of bacterial biofilm and the appearance of gingivitis within a period of 21 days in adults [10].

Gingivitis was confirmed to be reversible during the first 7 days if the discipline of adequate brushing to remove biofilm was restored; even when, from the beginning, the supragingival plaque had been largely dominated by gram-negative microorganisms, responsible for the aforementioned gingivitis [32].

Periodontal maintenance programs, which emphasize careful toothbrushing for adequate supragingival plaque control, reduce periodontal attachment loss in adults [32].

By way of conclusion, we can affirm the following:

1. The essential requirement for the prevention of a disease is to know its cause.

2. The high prevalence of the periodontal disease is proof of the insufficient capacity and security that we have to properly apply the knowledge acquired [33].

5. The dentist-educator

Dentists must understand that they need to assume the role of educators if they want to guarantee the success of periodontal treatment. It is not easy to get any change in the lifestyle of an adult. It is not easy to convince him of the urgency of change for a healthier life [33]. Someone said: "We all want a better life but to have a better life you have to be better." And that is only achieved by learning to change.

> *"Only someone who is devoted to a cause with all his might and soul can be a true teacher." – Einstein.*

There are numerous social and economic factors that are beyond the influence of the dentist, but even so, the profession has certain inalienable obligations: educate the patient about good oral hygiene habits, find ways to motivate him/her to apply the recommendations given, provide regular professional cleaning service (prophylaxis), apply fluoride to young teeth, use sealants, and, if the disease appears for collateral reasons, carry out a correct treatment that does not lead to damage or greater disease [33].

> *"It is not the strongest species that survives, nor the most intelligent, but the one that best responds to change." – Charles Darwin.*

The incorporation of the philosophy of prevention into ordinary work has to do with the way of thinking and disposition of each dentist [33].

Providing a preventive service, based on the active participation of the patient, suggests that even the word "patient" in that circumstance would be inappropriate, perhaps it would be better to qualify it and see it as a "student" [33].

The values and attitudes of the dentist do not necessarily coincide with those of the patient; he/she fundamentally wants to eat comfortably and look good. Instead, the clinician wants to achieve a zero-plaque score and a balanced occlusion. These different ways of approaching the success of the treatment have to be approached little by little, by conviction, because both are essential. The dentist must grade the information and give it in simple language, adapting to the level of understanding. He must generate such stimulation that the patient puts the instructions into practice because he/she has assumed the advantages of following them, as well as the disadvantages of ignoring them. Unfortunately, many dentists do not value this teaching task enough to give it their time or do not have sufficient preparation to tackle it, and even when faced with the advice to undertake it, they are impatient or arrogant [33].

Too often, dentists find it difficult to give themselves the space to provide patients with the necessary information or, sometimes, patients do not appreciate the value of the time spent instilling this valuable information in themselves [33].

As a didactic aid, we could say that the information should be enunciated based on a direct demonstration in the patient's own mouth, even better before starting treatment. It is very useful to provide the patient with a hand mirror so that he/she can observe part of the examination, point out the bacterial plaque and the calculus, and explain the relationship of these elements with periodontal disease.

Emphasize that bacterial plaque is the main cause of the disease. The plaque is almost always imperceptible, but by applying a revealing substance it becomes visible [33]. Once this is done, the patient is given a toothbrush and asked to try to remove all the stained plaques.

As a strategy, in such an instance, the patient should not be instructed in any particular brushing technique. Let the patient realize the difficulty he/she finds in completely removing bacterial plaque. This will make you more receptive to advise and reasons. When the patient becomes aware that it is very difficult for him/her to remove all the plaque, we will teach him/her a brushing technique and how he/she can develop the necessary skill [33].

The result of the patient's motivation and prophylactic education is not seen immediately, and it requires continued support by the dental staff, organized for this purpose, and the patient's perseverance [34].

Long-term studies conducted in Sweden by Axelsson and Lindhe provide convincing evidence of the benefits of a regular professional care program [35].

6. Tooth brushing requirements

1. The selected technique should clean all tooth surfaces, especially the gingival sulcus area and the interdental region.

2. Brushing should not injure hard or soft tissues.

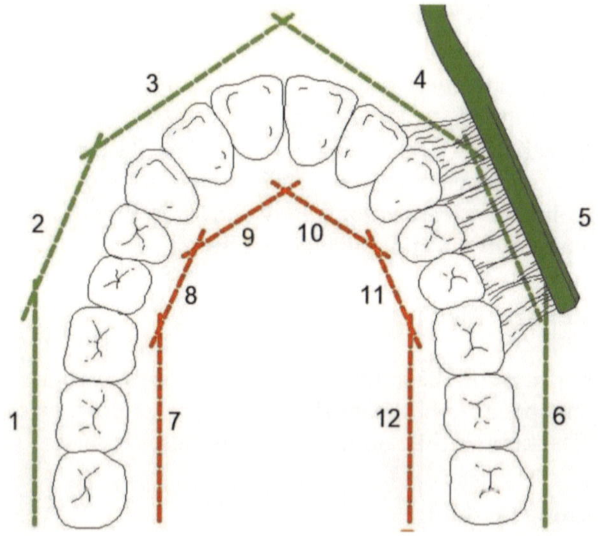

Figure 8.
If we divide each arch into 12 areas, we will achieve an orderly brushing that covers all the teeth. Adapted from MacPhee T., Cowley G [23].

3. The technique must be simple and easy to learn. An elementary technique for one patient may be difficult for another; therefore, each person needs to be guided in a personal way.

4. The technique must be organized through successive actions so that the entire dentition is brushed and no area is overlooked. For better systematization, it is advisable to divide the oral cavity into 12 sections [33] (**Figure 8**).

Each patient has different characteristics and, therefore, different needs, so there is no perfect brushing for all situations, but rather a brushing adapted to the individuality of the patient [36].

7. Oral hygiene methods

Several toothbrushing techniques have been proposed and recommended, including the following:

- Rubbing brushing method.
- Circular brushing method.
- Charters brushing method.
- Stillman brushing method.
- Bass brushing method.
- Electric brushing.

No brushing method has been shown to be superior to the rest [37].

7.1 Rubbing brushing method

It is perhaps the oldest [38]. Its brushing technique is the simplest, and it places the bristles on the teeth and moves back and forth. It does not require any prior training. The method is not aimed at cleaning the gingival margin. Vigorous rubbing with a stiff bristle brush can cause trauma and gingival recession.

7.2 Circular brushing method

The bristles are placed on the gums, and then, the brush is rotated over the surface of the teeth. On the upper teeth, the toothbrush is rotated downward. On the lower teeth, it goes up. The same is then done with the occlusal surfaces.

7.3 Charters planning method

The brush is directed toward the crown of the tooth, at an angle of 45°, in the opposite way to the Bass Technique [39].

7.4 Stillman planning method

The brush is directed at a 45° angle toward the gingiva and rotated toward the crown (twist technique) [39].

7.5 Bass technique

Dr. Charles Cassidy Bass, a medical doctor and researcher, described, in 1948, a dental brushing technique aimed at removing bacterial plaque from the gingival sulcus.

The brushing bristles are arranged so that there is an angle of approximately 45° relative to the long axis of the tooth. The brushing bristles should be directed toward the gingival sulcus. The brush is pressed against the gum and activated in a small circular motion so that the bristles enter the sulcus and are drawn into the sulcus area for cleaning. This action can be painful if the gingival tissues are inflamed and tender. It has been shown that it is the most effective method to remove bacterial plaque from the gingival area of the tooth. It is the method of choice also for healthy gums. The brush should have soft, rounded, and flexible bristles [40] (**Figures 9** and **10**).

In the following clinical case, it is possible to appreciate the efficiency of the Bass technique in the solution of a gingival inflammatory process. The patient is a 22-year-old university student (health sciences) who attended our private practice due to gingival bleeding for about 6 months. He had received dental care at a university clinic for several months and had seen no recovery from his periodontal health. Periodontal examination was performed. The periodontal diagnosis was as follows: chronic gingivitis and moderate gingival enlargement in some areas. The patient was very concerned about his periodontal health. It was explained to him that the first step to recovering his health was to develop a correct periodontal brushing technique to eliminate the biofilm, which causes chronic gingivitis. We detailed the Bass technique and he was given an appropriate brush. He also received information about the use of dental floss for interproximal areas, places where the brush cannot remove the biofilm.

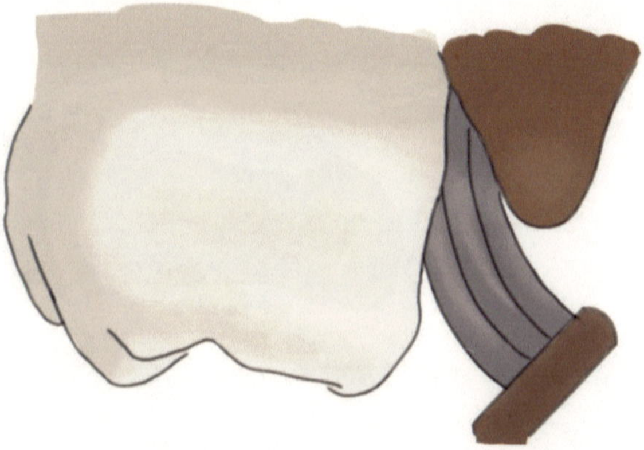

Figure 9.
Bass technique or sulcus brushing. The ends of the bristles are inserted into the gingival sulcus and over the marginal gingiva.

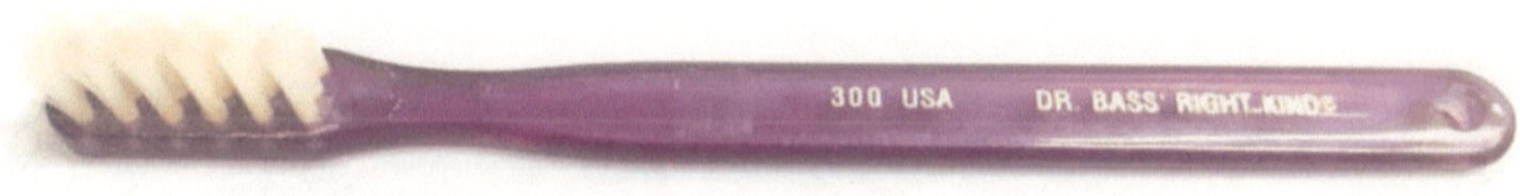

Figure 10.
The brush of Dr. Bass, pioneer of preventive dentistry, can now be found and purchased.

The dental assistant was in charge of biofilm control at each office visit. No other periodontal procedure such as scaling or root planning was applied. Only correct brushing was sufficient, during the period of periodontal treatment, to achieve absolute recovery of periodontal health (**Figures 1–20**).

7.6 Plate developer

They are substances capable of staining the bacterial biofilm to make it visible so that its removal is easier. Its application should be disseminated by all dentists since it allows locating where the biofilm is located and identifying the areas of the oral cavity

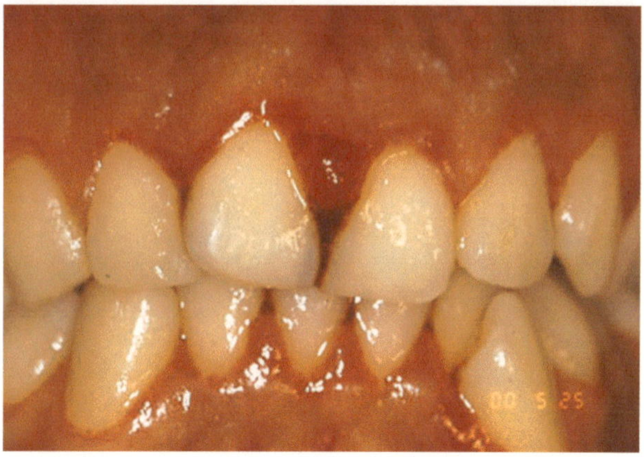

Figure 11.
On the first day of the consultation, it is noted that the patient has redness of the gingival margin, of the papillae and papillary enlargement. Spontaneous gingival bleeding may be noted.

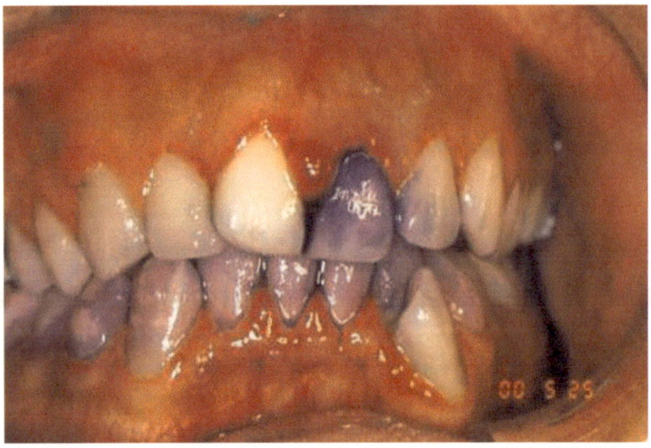

Figure 12.
The bacterial biofilm shows greater intensity and extension in the lower teeth. Lower dental crowding contributes to bacterial buildup.

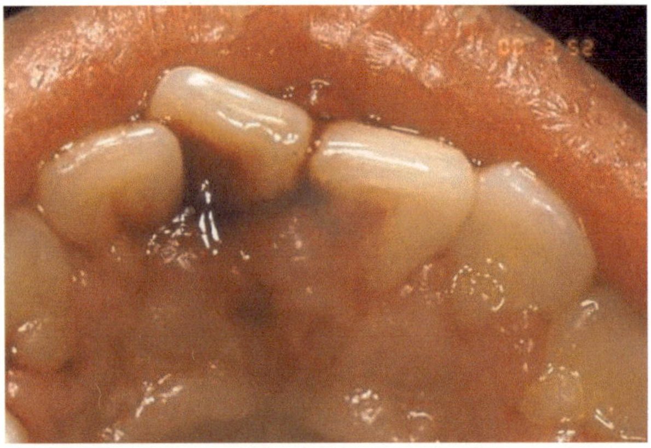

Figure 13.
Profuse and spontaneous gingival bleeding is observed on the palatal aspect of the maxillary anterior teeth. Dental crowding of the incisors contributes to this.

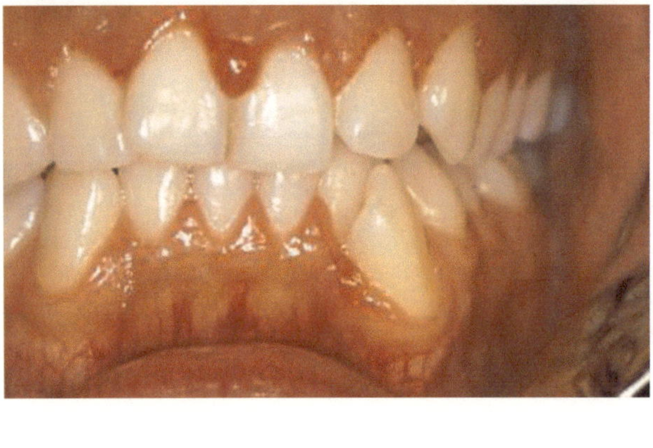

Figure 14.
After nine days of periodontal treatment with the application of the Bass technique, favorable gingival changes are manifested.

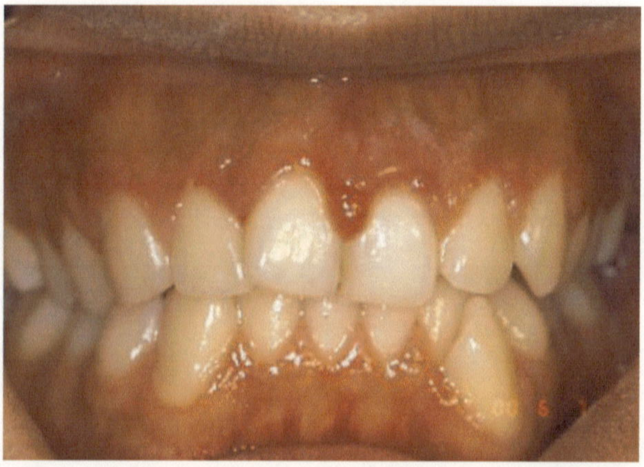

Figure 15.
After two weeks of treatment, the recovery of the patient's periodontal health is already noticeable.

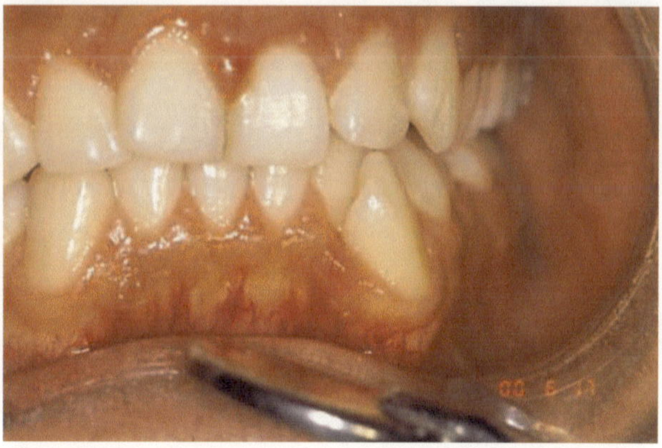

Figure 16.
At three weeks, the evolution of the periodontal treatment is very favorable. In the anterior and inferior regions, the periodontal tissues are completely healthy.

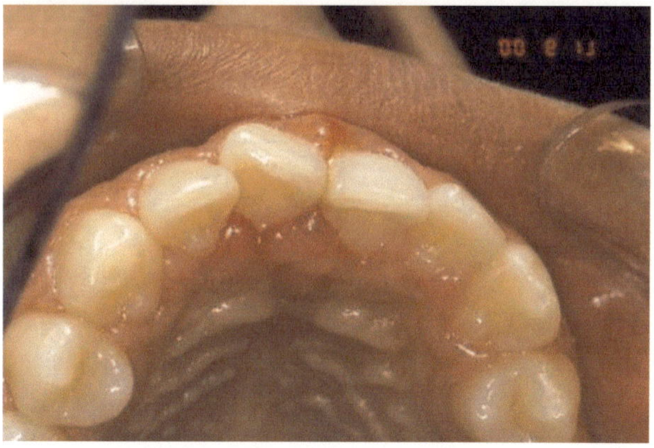

Figure 17.
After those three weeks of starting periodontal treatment, also the profuse gingival bleeding on the palatal aspects of the maxillary anterior teeth has ceased and the gingival papillae are healthier.

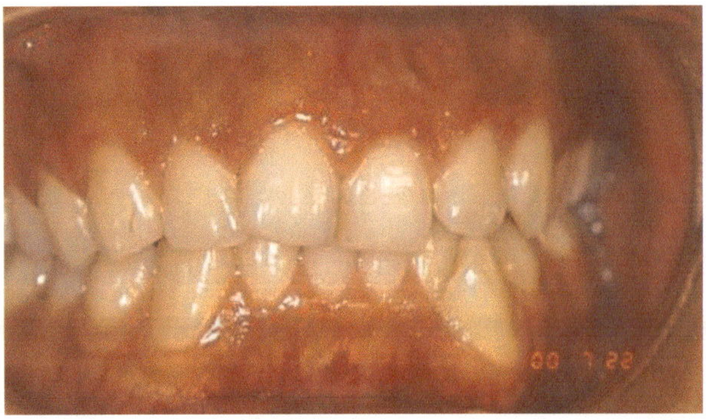

Figure 18.
Two months later, periodontal treatment with the Bass technique has restored 100% periodontal health.

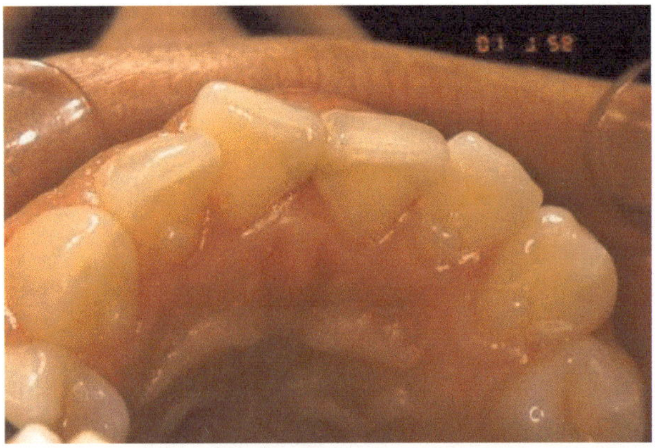

Figure 19.
After one year and two months of using the Bass technique and the use of dental floss, the periodontal tissues of the palatal surfaces continue to maintain their excellent periodontal health.

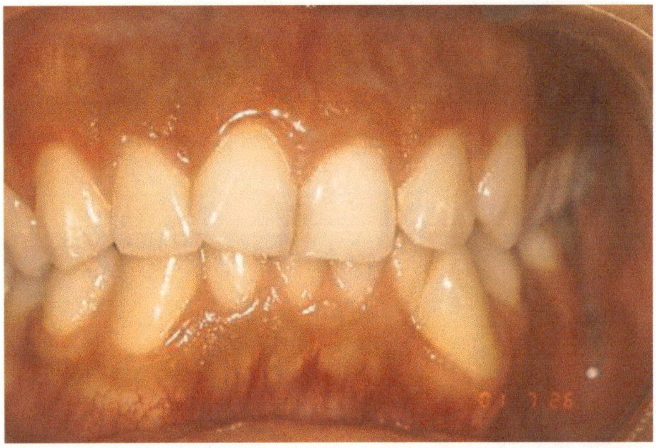

Figure 20.
In addition, after that year and two months, the periodontal tissues maintain their excellent periodontal health. If this disciplined care continues, the patient will enjoy an optimal quality of life, avoiding the appearance of periodontitis.

DOI: http://dx.doi.org/10.5772/intechopen.107332

that need more attention and better oral hygiene. The development of bacterial plaque or biofilm represents such an important step that it could be compared with periodontal diagnosis. Its use should be universal, even in periodontally healthy people. It is also a useful resource for choosing the most appropriate toothbrushing technique and recommending the use of dental floss. In this way, both dental caries and periodontal diseases are prevented.

Plaque or biofilm developers contain special dyes that stain biofilm red, pink, or purple. They come in pills, developer gel, developer liquid, and rinses. It is worth warning the patient that the staining will disappear with a well-executed brushing.

8. Dental floss

The interdental area is where biofilm, biofilm, or plaque is usually retained and, at the same time, the area most inaccessible to tooth brushing.

The most useful element to remove biofilm is dental floss because it is more effective than others. Its handling must be careful not to injure the interproximal gingiva. There is not much difference between flossing with wax or without wax.

A threader can be a good help in cleaning up hard-to-reach posterior areas. However, dental floss is currently manufactured with a special finish that allows it to be inserted comfortably in the posterior areas (**Figure 21**).

8.1 Technique of use of dental floss

1. The dental floss should be placed firmly around the knuckle of one finger of each hand. Then firmly hold a short portion between the guide fingers (**Figures** 22 and 23).

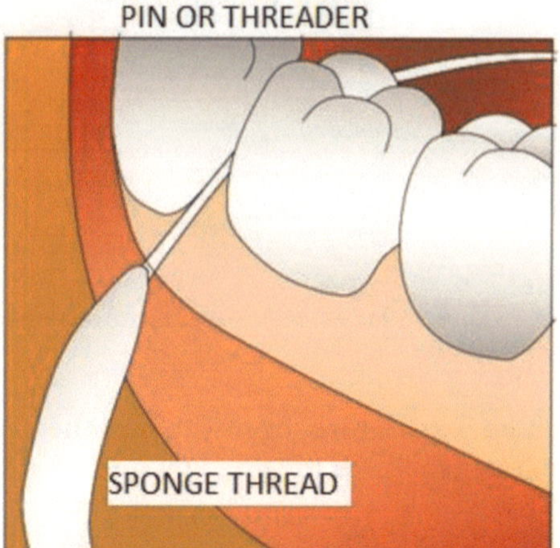

Figure 21.
Special dental floss with the following sections and characteristics: the first section, the threader, commonly the pin; second section, "sponge thread"; third and last section, standard dental floss.

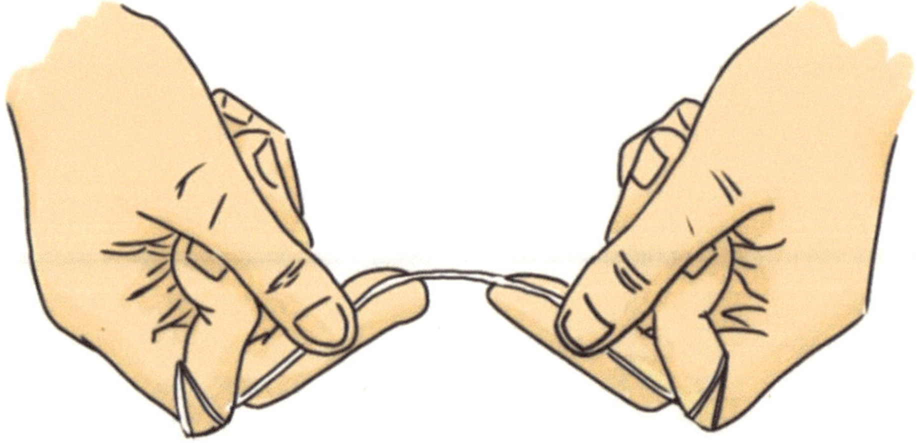

Figure 22.
An effective method of holding dental floss. Adapted from Pawlak EA and Hoag P.M [41].

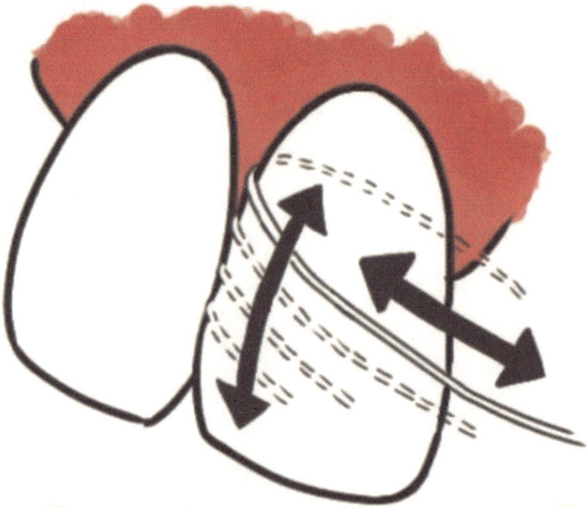

Figure 23.
Flossing. The wrapping around the vestibular and palatal (lingual) faces is to eliminate the largest amount of bacterial biofilm. Adapted from Pawlak EA and Hoag P.M [41].

1. The thread must not be forced, torn, or frayed past the point of contact. It should not damage the gingival papilla or the gingival sulcus.

2. The cord is placed at the base of the gingival sulcus and with gentle movements (down and up), and it should be brought from the sulcus to the interproximal contact point.

3. The dental floss moves along the tooth surface, not the gingival surface. The floss has to be curved around the tooth.

4. Dental floss must be used carefully, following the indicated technique, to avoid any trauma.

5. If the patient lacks the dexterity to use the thread properly, thread-holding devices will be recommended.

6. For bridges, it is suggested to use pins and special threads [41].

9. Special areas for oral hygiene

There are places or surfaces that are very difficult to clean, such as the following:

- Entrance of the forks.
- Concavities in distal areas of the molars, especially in case of root amputation.
- Any other place of the later pieces.
- Surfaces adjacent to edentulous areas.
- Areas adjacent to retention splints after orthodontics.

In these cases, the use of the single-plumed brush is very beneficial and favorable [42].

10. Other items for oral hygiene

Longitudinal studies reveal that sites with inadequate plaque removal have deeper probing depths and attachment loss after periodontal therapy [43, 44].

Some researchers recommend that the patient be instructed in the use of gauze pads as a good alternative to remove biofilm. The use of gauze is not traumatic.

It is advisable in special cases such as the following: after periodontal surgery, implant surgery, difficulty opening the mouth, lack of manual dexterity, disabled patients or patients with mobility problems. In addition, on surfaces adjacent to edentulous areas with the presence of crowns.

The gauze is recommended when food has been eaten apart from meal times or outside the home, and also if for some other reason when the toothbrush cannot be used [42]. The use of gauze in specialized clinics is very widespread to do the cleaning of the mucous membranes of the newborn after delivery (**Figures 24** and **25**).

The buccal, palatal or lingual, and occlusal surfaces of the teeth are easy to clean with toothbrushes, but these do not reach the interdental region of the teeth efficiently [45].

Slot DE et al., after a systematic review of the efficacy of manual brushes, reached the following conclusion: at the end of a brushing exercise, and only 42% of the biofilm is removed on average [46].

Other studies indicate that even using proper technique, you can clean only 65% of the total tooth surface. Due to the limitations of brushes in penetrating proximal areas and interdental hygiene, that is, flossing gains attention as a separate title. Interdental plaque biofilm control measures should consider perfecting tooth brushing so that it is a complement to mechanical cleaning [47, 48].

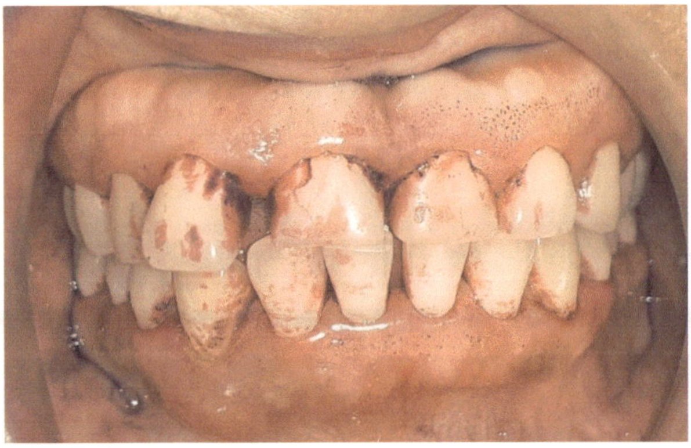

Figure 24.
A female patient diagnosed with chronic periodontitis III, grade A. Tooth separation and migration of tooth 1.2 is evident.

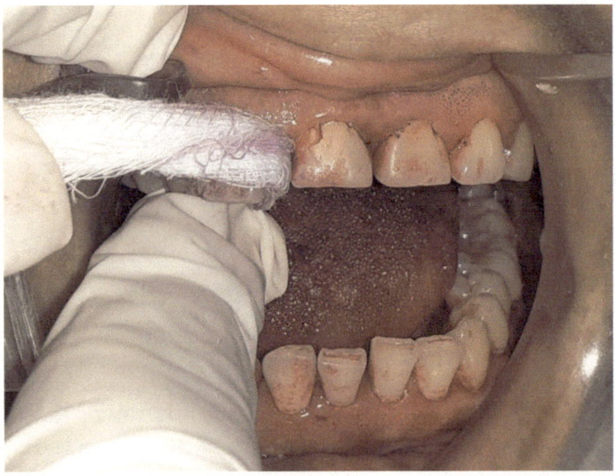

Figure 25.
As an alternative, given the area, to remove the biofilm between teeth 1.2 and 1.1, the patient can use gauze.

Since patients have different types of dentition and also different interdental spaces, it will be advisable to recommend the appropriate devices according to the individuality of the patient, and also guide him/her in considering his/her personal needs [48].

Added to this is that patients pay more attention to the anterior areas and brush the posterior teeth very superficially on their palatal and lingual surfaces.

For the maintenance of periodontal health and the prevention of dental caries, tooth brushing should be combined with interdental cleaning once every 24 hours [49, 50].

A recent study, conducted on young subjects without interdental attachment loss, found that toothbrushing, in combination with dental flossing, is capable of reducing both plaque and gingival inflammation [51].

When the interdental space is filled with the gingival papilla, especially in the case of young people, dental floss is the best option to reach this area [52].

Christo et al. designed a randomized, split-mouth clinical trial that aimed to compare the clinical efficacy of flossing and interdental brushing, along with tooth brushing. After 6 weeks, in combination with a manual toothbrush, interdental brushing was found to be more effective in removing plaque and reducing probing depth compared to flossing [53].

On the way to the definitive solution, it is an excellent support to educate patients on prevention measures, trying to be more explicit and insistent with those who do not have dental insurance. Thus, gradually, they will alleviate their periodontal diseases and achieve optimal dental health.

> *"In the long history of humanity and also of the animal world, those who learned to collaborate and improvise are the ones who have prevailed." Charles Darwin [54].*

Patients may know and understand the benefits of flossing and rinsing, but only 1 in 6 make them a daily habit. These good practices are not widely executed by the general population. Among the barriers experienced by the respondents we have: fear of bleeding, gingival pain, and forgetting to floss or rinse in their daily hygiene despite knowing that these habits would improve their oral health [55].

The critical problem for clinicians is not the arrest of periodontal disease, but rather the identification of patients at high risk of experiencing the active and progressive disease. This challenge raises the issue that perhaps dentistry needs to change its approach to gum disease [56].

11. Conclusion

Bacterial biofilm is the main etiological agent of periodontal diseases. Periodontal diseases can be prevented with simple procedures: good brushing technique and use of dental floss. The removal of bacterial biofilm with regular brushing is efficient, but it is not enough. The complementation with other hygiene elements (interdental brushes, dental floss, gauze, mouth rinses, interdental rubber bristles, oral irrigator, and others) achieves excellent results, as demonstrated by many research works. Dentists and auxiliary personnel must assume their roles in a leading role, and become aware of their responsibility in the prevention of periodontal diseases wherever they have to practice.

> *"What would life be if we didn't have the courage to try something new?"*
> *Vincent Van Gogh.*

Acknowledgements

To Professor Mag. Lily Cardich for her thorough revision of her style from the original manuscript. To Ms. Karime Z. Salas Garcia for her illustrations for the article, as well as her great responsibility. Likewise, to Ms. Nuria L. Salas Garcia for her diligent work in typing the original document.

Conflict of interest

"The authors declare no conflict of interest."

Author details

Luis V. Maita-Véliz* and Luis M. Maita-Castañeda
National University of San Marcos, Lima, Peru

*Address all correspondence to: lmaitav@unmsm.edu.pe

References

[1] Page RC, Kornman KS. The pathogenesis of human periodontitis: An introduction. Periodontology 2000. 1997;**14**:9-11. DOI: 10.1111/j.1600-0757.1997.tb00189.x

[2] Page RC, Offenbacher S, Schroeder HE, Seymour GJ, Kornman KS. Advances in the pathogenesis of periodontitis: Summary of developments, clinical implications and future directions. Periodontology 2000. 1997;**14**:48-216. DOI: 10.1111/j.1600-0757.1997.tb00199.x

[3] Cobb CM. Non-surgical pocket therapy: Mechanical. Annals of Periodontology. 1996;**1**(1):90-443. DOI: 10.1902/annals.1996.1.1.443

[4] Dentino A, Lee S, Mailhot J, et al. Principles of periodontology. Periodontology 2000. 2013;**61**(1):16-53. DOI: 10.1111/j.1600-0757.2011.00397.x

[5] Claydon N, Addy M. Comparative single-use plaque removal by toothbrushes of different designs. Journal of Clinical Periodontology. 1996;**23**(12):6-1112

[6] Egelberg J, Claffey N. Consensus report: The role of mechanical dental plaque removal in prevention and therapy of caries and periodontal diseases. In: Proceedings of the European Workshop of Mechanical Plaque Control. Chicago, Quintessence. 1998. pp. 169-172

[7] Der Weijden V, f, Slot DE. Oral hygiene in the prevention of periodontal diseases: The evidence. Periodontol. 2011;**55**:104-123

[8] Morillo M, González Y. Plan motivacional para la formación del hábito de higiene bucal en los pacientes que asisten a la clínica integral del adulto del área de odontología de la Universidad Nacional Experimental Rómulo Gallegos. Acta Odontológica Venezolana. 2018;**46**(1):56-60

[9] Roncati M. Terapia periodontal no quirúrgica. España: Editorial Quintessence S.R. Barcelona; 2016

[10] Löe H, Theilade E, Jensen SB. Experimental gingivitis in man. Journal of Periodontology. 1965;**36**:87-177

[11] Suomi JD, Green JC, Vermillion J, et al. The effect of controlled oral hygiene procedures on the progression of periodontal disease in adults: Results after two years. Journal of Periodontology. 1969;**40**(7):416-420

[12] De la Rosa M, Guerra JZ, Johnston DA, et al. Plaque growth and removal with daily toothbrushing. Journal of Periodontology. 1979;**50**(12):661-664

[13] Hellström MK, Ramberg P, Krok L, et al. The effects of supragingival plaque control on the subgingival microflora in human periodontitis. Journal of Clinical Periodontology. 1996;**23**(10):40-934

[14] Straub AM, Salvi GE, Lang NP. Supragingival plaque formation in the human dentition. In: Lang NP, Ättstrom R, Löe H, editors. Proceedings of the European Workshop on Mechanical Plaque Control. Chicago: Quintessence; 1998

[15] Greenwell H. Committee on research, science and therapy. American academy of periodontology. position paper: Guidelines for periodontal therapy. Journal of Periodontology. 2001;**72**(11):8-1624

[16] Kinane DF. The role of interdental cleaning in effective plaque control: Need for interdental cleaning in primary and secondary prevention. In: Lang NP, Ättstrom R, Löe H, editors. Proceedings of the European Workshop on Mechanical Plaque Control. Chicago: Quintessence; 1998

[17] Teles RP, Patel M, Socransky SS, et al. Disease progression in periodontally healthy and maintenance subjects. Journal of Periodontology. 2008;**79**(5):94-784

[18] Grossman E, Reiter G, Sturzenberg OP, et al. Six-month study of the effects of a chlorhexidine mouthrinse on gingivitis in adults. Journal of Periodontal Research. 1986;**21** (Suppl):33-43

[19] Bascones A, Morante S, Mateos L, et al. Influence of additional active ingredients on the effectiveness of non-alcoholic chlorhexidine mouthwashes: A randomized controlled trial. Journal of Periodontology. 2005;**76**(9):75-1469

[20] Ramos Perfecto D, Maita VL. Tratamiento de la periodontitis en pacientes diabéticos tipo 2 mediante el uso de oleorresina de copaiba como coadyuvante. In: Centro de Producción Imprenta Editorial de la Universidad Nacional Mayor de San Marcos. 2019

[21] Ramos Perfecto D, Maita Véliz L, Maita Castañeda ML, Castro LA. Un producto natural de posible apoyo al tratamiento de la periodontitis: Revisión bibliográfica. Avances en Odontoestomatologia. 2020;**36**(3): 143-149

[22] Ciancio SG. Chemical agents: Plaque control, calculus reduction and treatment of dentinal hypersensitivity. Periodontology 2000. 1995;**8**:7-136

[23] Mac Phee T, Cowley G. Essencials of Periodontology and Periodontics. Second ed. Oxford: Blackwell Scientific Publicactions Osney Mead; 1975

[24] Drisko CL. Periodontal self-care: Evidence-based support. Periodontology 2000. 2013;**62**(1):55-243

[25] Khocht A, Simon G, Person P, et al. Gingival recession in relation to history of hard toothbrush use. Journal of Periodontology. 1993;**64**(9):5-900

[26] Agudio G, Pini Prato GP, Cortellini P. Gingival lesions due to improper methods of oral hygiene. Mondo Odontostomatologico. 1984; **26**(3):45-53

[27] Danser MM, Timmerman MF, Ijzerman Y, et al. Evaluation of the incidence of gingival abrasion as a result of toothbrushing. Journal of Clinical Periodontology. 1998;**25**(9): 6-701

[28] Silverstone LM, Featherstone MJ. A scanning electron microscope study of the end rounding of bristles in eight toothbrush types. Quintessence International. 1988;**19**(2):87-107

[29] Bass CC. The optimum characteristics of toothbrushes for personal oral hygiene. Dental Items of Interest. 1948;**70**(7):697-718

[30] West NX, Moran JM. Home-use preventive and therapentic oral products. Periodontology 2000. 2008; **48**:7-9

[31] Pattison GA. Self-inflicted gingival injuries: Literature review and case report. Journal of Periodontology. 1983; **54**(5):299-304

[32] Axelsson P, Lindhe J. Effect of controlled oral hygiene procedures on

caries and periodontal disease in adults. Journal of Clinical Periodontology. 1978; **5**(2):133-151

[33] Eley BM, Soory M, MJD. Periodoncia. Sexta edición ed. España: Elsevier; 2012. pp. 152-162

[34] Sims W. Preventive dentistry for the dental practitioner. Dental Practice. 1968;**18**:309-314

[35] Axelsson P, Lindhe J. The effect of a preventive programme on dental plaque, gingivitis and caries in schoolchildren. Results after one and two years. Journal of Clinical Periodontology. 1974;**1**(2): 126-138

[36] Bascones MA. Periodoncia Clínica e Implantologia Oral. 4ta edición. 2014. Ediciones Avances Médico-Dentales, España, S.L

[37] Raposa K. Oral infections control: Toothbrushes and toothbrushing. In: Wilkins EM, editor. Clinical Practice of the Dental Hygienist. 11th ed. Philadelphia, PA: Lippincott Willians & Wilkins; 2013. pp. 389-407

[38] Perry DA, Beemsterboer PL, Essex G. Periodontología para el higienista dental. Cuarta edición. 2014 Elsevier España, S.L

[39] Müller HP. Periodontología. México: Editorial El Manual Moderno; 2006

[40] Manson JD. Manual de Periodoncia. Editorial El Manual Moderno, S.A de C.V; 1986

[41] Pawlak EA, y Hoag PM. Conceptos esenciales de periodoncia, 1ra. Editorial Mundi S.A.I.C. y F. 1978

[42] Roncati M. Terapia periodontal no quirúrgica. España: Editorial Quintessence L.L; 2016

[43] Jackson MA, Kellett M, Worthington HV, Clerehugh V. Comparison of interdental cleaning methods: A randomized controlled trial. Journal of Periodontology. 2006;**77**(8): 1421-1429

[44] Loos B, Nylund K, Claffey N, Egelberg J. Clinical effects of root debridement in molar and nonmolar teeth. A 2 year follow-up. Journal of Clinical Periodontology. 1989;**16**(8):498-504

[45] Caton JG, Blieden TM, Lowenguth RA, Frantz BJ, Wagener CJ, Doblin JM, et al. Comparison between mechanical cleaning and an antimicrobial rinse for the treatment and prevention of interdental gingivitis. Journal of Clinical Periodontology. 1993; **20**(3):172-178

[46] Solt DE, Wiggelinkhuisen L, Rosema NA, Van der Weijden GA. The efficacy of manual toothbrushes following a brushing exercise: A systematic review. International Journal of Dental Hygiene. 2012;**10**(3):187-197

[47] Lang NP, Cumming BR, Löe HA. Oral hygiene and gingival health in Danish dental students and faculty. Community Dentistry and Oral Epidemiology. 1977;**5**(5):237-242

[48] Sälzer S, Slot DE, Van der Weijden FA, Dörfer CE. Efficacy of inter-dental mechanical plaque control in managing gingivitis–A meta-review. Journal of Clinical Periodontology. 2015; **42**(Suppl 16):S92-S105

[49] Lang NP, Cumming BR, Löe H. Toothbrushing frequency as it relates to plaque development and gingival health. Journal of Periodontology. 1973;**44**(7): 396-405

[50] Axelsson P, Nyström B, Lindhe J. The long-term effect of a plaque control

program on tooth mortality, caries and periodontal disease in adults. Results after 30 years of maintenance. Journal of Clinical Periodontology. 2004;**31**(9): 749-757

[51] Graziani F, Palazzolo A, Gennai S, Karapetsa D, Giuca MR, Cei S, et al. Interdental plaque reduction after use of different devices in young subjects with intact papilla: A randomized clinical trial. International Journal of Dental Hygiene. 2018;**16**(3):389-396

[52] Schmage P, Platzer U, Nergiz I. Comparison between manual and mechanical methods of interproximal hygiene. Quintessence International. 1999;**30**(8):535-539

[53] Christou V, Timmerman MF, Van der Velden U, Van der Weijden FA. Comparison of different approaches of interdental oral hygiene: Interdental brushes versus dental floss. Journal of Periodontology. 1998;**69**(7):759-764

[54] Carlos Román-Mateo y Raul Delgado-Morales. Genética y evolución. Pasado y futuro de nuestros genes. El futuro de la Humanidad. National geographic. RBA Editores México. Capítulo 04. Página 113 2019

[55] Rotella K et al. Habits, practices and beliefs regarding floss and mouthrinse among habitual and non-habituals users. Journal of Dental Hygiene. 2022;**96**(3): 46-58

[56] Gellibolian R et al. Precision periodontics. Quantitave measures of disease progression. The Journal of Dryland Agriculture. 2022:**153**(9): 826-828

Chapter 8

Advances in Locally Delivered Antimicrobials for Periodontitis Treatment

Irina-Georgeta Sufaru, Maria-Alexandra Martu, Ionut Luchian, Silvia Teslaru, Simona Stoleriu, Stefan-Ioan Stratul, Darian Rusu, Monica Silvia Tatarciuc and Sorina Mihaela Solomon

Abstract

Periodontal disease represents an inflammatory disease of the tissues supporting the maintenance and functionality of the teeth on the dental arches. The main cause of periodontitis consists in periodontal dysbiosis, which will trigger an inflammatory response, progressively leading to periodontal tissue breakdown. Scaling and root planing represent the gold standard in treating periodontal diseases but, as it was already established, these measures are unable to completely eliminate the subgingival bacterial plaque. Therefore, new adjunctive therapies have emerged, involving systemic and local delivery of various antimicrobial products. This chapter aims to provide current knowledge on the local application of different periodontal supplementary therapies. The chapter focuses on local forms of antimicrobials, such as irrigations, gels or controlled release systems but also on laser/LED-assisted periodontal pocket photodynamic antibacterial therapy (PDT), along with various photosensitizers. Moreover, we present data from current guidelines regarding the recommendations for the main locally delivered antimicrobials.

Keywords: antimicrobials, local adjunctive periodontal therapy, periodontitis, photodynamic antibacterial therapy, photosensitizer

1. Introduction

Periodontal disease is an immuno-inflammatory condition that affects periodontal tissues, caused by multifactorial etiologies [1]. The disease is the result of complex interactions between periodontopathogenic bacteria, organized in biofilm, and the host's immune response; the latter is considered to account for almost 80% of the risk [2].

In periodontal health, there is a balance between the microbial flora and the host's immune system. Disrupting this balance will trigger an immune response, activating the mechanisms of innate and adaptive immunity. Periodontal pathogens generate a number of products that will cause the destruction of the extracellular matrix, as well as increase the permeability of the host cell membranes, leading to a subsequent tissue invasion [3]. Among the most aggressive periodontal pathogens are *Porphyromonas gingivalis*, *Tannerella forsythia*, *Treponema denticola*, *Prevotella intermedia* or *Aggregatibacter actinomycetemcomitans* [4].

Following the interaction between the pathogenic flora and the immune system, the release of proinflammatory molecules takes place, molecules that will exacerbate the inflammatory status, with the subsequent appearance, over time, of periodontal attachment loss and the progressive deep invasion of pathogens and their products [5]. If proper periodontal therapy is not instituted, the disease can have unfavorable consequences, such as the occurrence of dental hypersensitivity, dental mobility, pathological dental migration and, ultimately, tooth loss. Moreover, the complications of periodontal disease can extend to systemic level, exacerbating already established conditions such as diabetes, rheumatoid arthritis or cardiovascular diseases [6]. Factors that can affect the appearance and evolution of periodontitis can be both local (poor oral hygiene, dental malposition, incorrect prosthetic or orthodontic treatments) and general; the latter include modifiable factors, such as lifestyle, certain drugs or even systemic pathologies, but also non-modifiable factors (genetic, epigenetic factors or uncontrollable diseases) [7].

The first step in periodontal treatment includes addressing the factors that led to the onset and development of periodontal disease. This particular phase of treatment includes periodontal scaling and root planing (SRP) which are, to date, the therapeutical gold standard, which cannot be replaced by other therapeutic means. SRP aims to disorganize the periodontal biofilm and create "biologically acceptable" areas and surfaces, which would allow healing and obtaining the status of "periodontal health" [8].

The major disadvantage of SRP is its inefficiency in periodontal pockets with complex anatomies, where access is difficult or even impossible; thus, adjunctive, systemic or local antibacterial therapies are sometimes required. Systemic antibiotic therapy, however, is accompanied by a number of less favorable characteristics, such as hepatic or renal toxicity, the risk of gastrointestinal complications, the appearance of resistant microorganisms or poor biodistribution in sites of interest [9]. Thus, a favorable alternative is the local administration of therapeutic, antimicrobials or anti-inflammatory agents, in various forms of administration. Pharmacological agents placed directly in the periodontal pocket can generate an adequate concentration for a sufficiently long period of time, without systemic complications and with improved patient compliance [10]. Below we will present the main local forms of antibacterial drug therapy.

2. Classification of local antibacterial therapy systems

Local forms of antibacterial drug therapy can be used either at home, by the patient or in the dental office, is considered professional methods. They can also be classified as nonsustained, sustained or controlled release systems (**Figure 1**).

Nonsustained release systems are characterized by the immediate release of the active agent, without in situ retention; these systems usually include supra- and sub-gingival irrigation solutions. In the case of sustained release devices, a high concentration of chemotherapeutic agent is obtained in the periodontal pocket for an extended period; this is the case with varnishes or gels. These forms of therapy can also be applied at home, but absolutely require a good knowledge of the application technique by the patient.

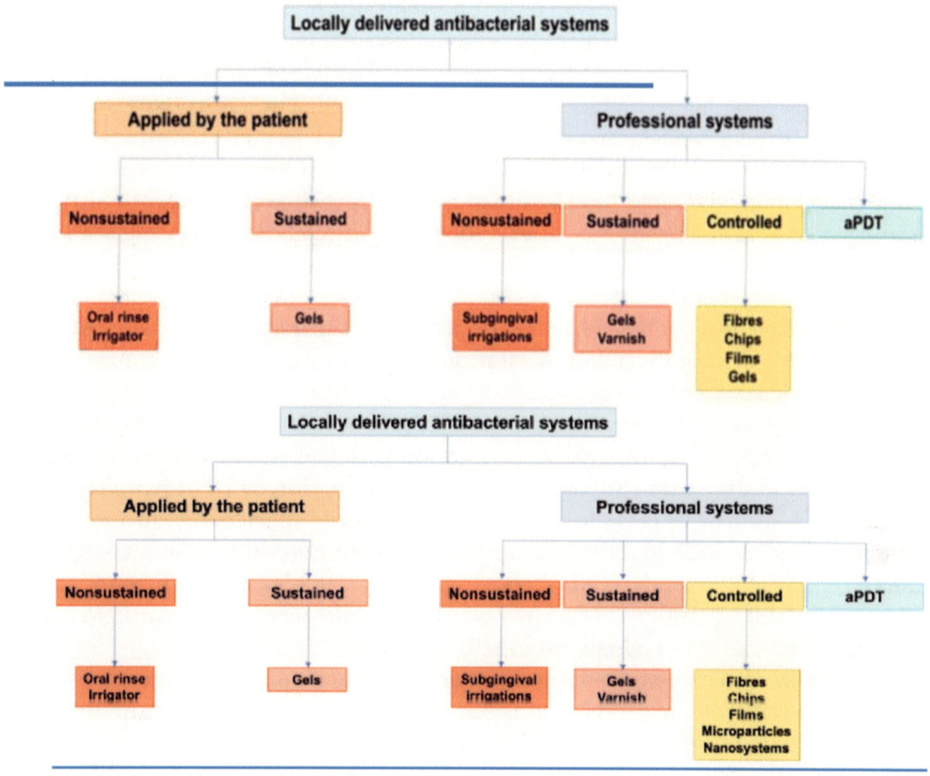

Figure 1.
Classification of locally delivered antibacterial systems.

Controlled-release systems include fibers, chips, films or certain gels that contain the active substance in the delivery medium and are placed in the periodontal pocket by a specialist in the dental office; they will slowly release adequate concentrations of the active substance over a period longer than 24 hours.

A potentially efficient method involves the photodynamic antibacterial therapy of periodontal pockets, which involves the application of light radiation (laser or LED), often together with a photosensitizing substance.

3. Irrigation solutions

Irrigation systems usually involve the use of a cannula connected to a syringe containing solutions of various active substances, such as chlorhexidine, triclosan, povidone-iodine, ozonated water or even sodium hypochlorite [11]. Bacteria and their products can be eliminated by the constant pressure of the solution on the tissue, along with drug activity [12].

The obtained data generally indicate that these irrigation solutions may lead to a number of improvements in periodontal parameters (plaque index, bleeding index on probing, depth on probing or periodontal clinical attachment loss), but these benefits appear to be in the short-term [13–16]. The main explanation for this phenomenon is given by the transient action of the active substance which is easily washed from the site by the action of saliva and crevicular fluid.

Chlorhexidine concentrations in irrigation solutions investigated in clinical trials range from 0.02% to 0.2%. The data provided, however, indicate that they do not bring an additional benefit over SRP alone [17, 18]. The use of povidone-iodine generated a minimal probing depth reduction of 0.28 mm [19]. The use of 0.5% sodium hypochlorite in subgingival irrigation did not generate unwanted side effects but also no additional periodontal benefit [20]. Da Costa et al. [21] performed a systematic review that evaluated the use of chlorhexidine mouthwash as an adjunct to SRP for chronic periodontitis. The authors observed that additional mouth rinsing with chlorhexidine resulted in slightly greater probing depth reduction than SRP alone, a negligible effect on clinical attachment level and potential for tooth staining [21].

An interesting approach is the use of desiccants in the irrigation of periodontal pockets. These are generally aqueous solutions of a mixture of hydroxybenzenesulfonic and hydroxymethoxybenzenesulfonic and sulfuric acid, which have a hygroscopic surface and a denaturing action [22]. These solutions have the ability to dehydrate the bacterial biofilm matrix. Irrigation with Hybenx®, a mixture of sulfonated phenols, additional to SRP, generated, after evaluation by DNA pyrosequencing, the elimination of 13 periodontopathogenic bacterial species [23]. In another study by Isola et al., SRP adjuvant therapy with Hybenx® resulted in more significant reductions in probing depth, clinical attachment loss and bleeding on probing, as well as red complex pathogens (*Porphyromonas gingivalis, Treponema denticola* and *Tannerella forsythia*) when compared to SRP alone [24].

Recently, we also investigated the effect of probiotic irrigation solutions (*Lactobacillus reuteri* DSM 17938); results at 3 months indicated significant improvements in periodontal attachment and bleeding on probing [25].

Therefore, the data in the literature on irrigation solutions are quite heterogeneous and, to date, there is no information to support the long-term effectiveness of these methods. Due to these limitations of subgingival irrigation solutions, their use is not a reliable method of professional control of bacterial plaque.

4. Varnishes

Varnishes used in periodontal treatments are generally based on chlorhexidine. Commercially available preparations include: Cervitec® Plus (Ivoclar/Vivadent AG, Schaan, Liechtenstein), with 1% chlorhexidine and 1% thymol in a polyvinyl butyral viscous base; EC40® (Biodent BV, Nijmegen, The Netherlands), solution of 35% chlorhexidine diacetate in 37% alcohol base stabilized with 27% sandarac; BioC® (Biodent BV, Nijmegen, The Netherlands), the supersaturated concentration of 20% chlorhexidine diacetate [26].

All these products have shown improvements in periodontal destruction rates but also reductions in bacterial load [27–30].

5. Gels

Gels are perhaps one of the most commonly used sustained release systems due to their ease of application, with the aid of cannula syringes and wide availability. Periodontal gels can be found in ready-made, available as commercial products (Chlo-Site®, Elyzol®, Atridox®, Periocline) or as pharmacy/laboratory products.

The active substances include chlorhexidine, triclosan or antibiotics, such as tetracycline, doxycycline, metronidazole or azithromycin, but also phytotherapeutic products such as curcumin or propolis. These substances are found in various polymer-based formulas, including xanthan, carbopol or chitosan.

Chlo-Site® is a gel containing 1.5% chlorhexidine in a xanthan matrix; it dissolves in 10–30 days after application, with an in situ therapeutic concentration maintained for 15 days, on average [12]. This prolonged release is possible because the matrix is mucoadhesive, which prevents it from being washed by saliva or GCF. In a systematic review, Tan et al. observed a 0.56 mm reduction in probing depth and a 0.53 mm periodontal attachment gain following the application of this gel [26]. Overall, the data support an additional beneficial effect of chlorhexidine gel application over SRP alone [31, 32].

Atridox® is a bi-component system, a 10% doxycycline hydrochloride thixotropic gel; it solidifies on contact with GCF. Studies have shown that doxycycline levels can remain above 1000 μg/mL for 18 hours in GCF, after which they begin to gradually decrease [33]. The doxycycline-based gel is effective as adjunctive therapy to SRP in terms of both clinical [34, 35] and microbiological parameters [36].

Minocycline 2% is found in biodegradable preparations with hydroxyethyl cellulose matrix, aminoalkyl methacrylate, triacetin and glycerin, such as Dentomycin® and Periocline®. In a study by van Steenberghe et al., the concentration of minocycline in GCF reached 1300 μg/mL at 1 hour but decreased to 90 μg/mL after 7 hours [37]. A minocycline and poly lactic-co-glycolic acid/N-methyl-pyrrolidone gel was developed, with favorable periodontal clinical results [38].

Metronidazole gel (Elyzol®) is a compound that becomes viscous on contact with GCF, which contains 40% metronidazole benzoate in an oil-based mixture (glyceryl monooleate and sesame oil), which is slowly broken down by GCF enzymes in 25% metronidazole [26, 39]. Data from the literature also support the efficacy of this preparation in combination with SRP, without the occurrence of systemic side effects [39–41].

Beneficial results were also obtained after applying 0.5% azithromycin [42], 0.4% moxifloxacin [43] or 3% satranidazole gels [44].

Another therapeutic option is given by deeply eutectic antimicrobial gels, such as choline and geranate gel (CAGE). Nakajima et al. demonstrated in a CAGE in vitro and in vivo study deep tissue penetration and antimicrobial activity against *P. gingivalis* [45].

Phytotherapeutic products, such as propolis [46] or turmeric [47], have also been addressed in the development of gels with subgingival application. Dave et al. observed significant reductions in plaque index, bleeding on probing, probing depth and periodontal clinical attachment loss after turmeric gel [48]. The 21-day application of turmeric gel versus chlorhexidine gel also showed significant reductions in plaque and gingival index, similar for both substances [49]; it should be noted, however, that turmeric gel was more easily tolerated by patients than chlorhexidine gel, the latter causing a bitter taste and pigmentation. The application of turmeric gel has also generated significant reductions in periodontal pathogens [50, 51].

6. Microparticle systems

Microparticles (microspheres) are solid, spherical polymeric structures with a diameter of 1–1000 μm, uniformly dispersed in a polymer matrix [2]. They contain active substances, generally antibiotics such as tetracycline, minocycline, doxycycline, metronidazole or clindamycin [11]. Microspheres can be made of resorbable and non-resorbable materials. The material of choice in their manufacturing remains, however, poly lactic-co-glycolic acid, due to its stability and the possibility of adjusting the released dose [2].

Arestin® (OraPharma, Inc., Warminster, PA, USA), a minocycline-based product, was approved by the FDA in 2001; it is presented as a single-dose cartridge, with 4 mg of bioresorbable microspheres of poly lactic-co-glycolic acid, with a diameter of 20–60 μm [26]. This powdered product hydrolyzes on contact with the crevicular fluid and provides a minocycline concentration of 340 μg/mL for 14 days [52]. Numerous studies support the clinical and microbiological efficacy of this product in patients with periodontitis, with and without systemic risk conditions [53–55].

Doxycycline-based products were also studied, with very favorable results. It has also been shown that a high concentration of doxycycline in the periodontal pocket was maintained for 20 days [56]. Ali et al. demonstrated, by developing a double emulsion system of microspheres of poly lactic-co-glycolic acid and doxycycline, a significant reduction of *P. gingivalis* and *Fusobacterium nucleatum* pathogens [57]. Clinically significant improvements and reductions in *P. gingivalis* have also been observed with the combination of doxycycline with metronidazole, encapsulated in solid lipid microparticles [58]. Wang et al. investigated the incorporation of bioactive agents into polylactic-co-glycolic acid microspheres dispersed in a thermo-reversible polyisocyanopeptide hydrogel; doxycycline and lipoxin were charged separately in acid-terminated and ester-coated polylactic-co-glycolic acid [59]. According to the authors, this system showed adequate injectability as well as long-term structural stability; in addition, no inflammatory response has been reported in vivo [59].

Very good results were also observed after the use of microspheres with tetracycline [12] or clindamycin [60].

7. Nanosystems

Nanosystems include products in the form of nanoparticles, nanofibers, mycelium or liposomes. These are systems that are still in the research phase, and no commercial products are available so far. Nanoparticles include nanospheres and nanocapsules in the solid state, amorphous or crystalline, with a diameter of about 10–200 nm [11].

The major advantage of these systems, in addition to their biocompatibility, is the ability of the product to reach less accessible sites, precisely because of the very small size of the particles, and can penetrate even the attachment epithelium [61]. Moreover, the high ratio between surface area and volume characteristic of these systems favors the loading with the active substance, reducing the frequency of application [2].

Although the concept of nanoparticles is not new in dentistry, the focus on loading them with antimicrobial substances has received relatively recent attention. PEG-PLA nanoparticles with minocycline have been shown to have prolonged-release properties, in effective concentrations and with improvements in periodontal parameters [61]. Another study evaluated the biocompatibility and antibacterial capacity of chitosan nanoparticles with doxycycline [62]; the authors showed that 50 nm particles showed approximately 75% capture efficiency and 28% loading capacity, good cellular compatibility, as well as antibacterial and anti-inflammatory activity [62].

Liposomes are microscopic vesicles based on lipids, unilamellar or multilamellar. Liposomes are produced from cholesterol, long-chain fatty acids, non-toxic surfactants, sphingolipids, glycolipids and membrane proteins [11]. The advantages of these products include biocompatibility, good distribution, stability, biodegradation capacity, as well as protection of the active substance against environmental factors [63]. Liu & Yang demonstrated, in a murine model of periodontitis, the efficiency of liposomes with minocycline 2% on both periodontal parameters and TNF-α [64]. The main disadvantage is the high production cost, along with the complexity of their realization and the still high degree of instability. However, liposome-based systems can be a promising direction in adjunctive periodontal therapy.

8. Fibers

Fibers represent carrier systems made of different materials, impregnated with the active substance. They are placed circumferentially in the periodontal pocket and may or may not be sealed with acrylic cements to keep them in place.

Actisite® is perhaps the best-known fibers system; it consists of non-resorbable fibers impregnated with 25% g/g tetracycline, equivalent to 12.7 mg tetracycline hydrochloride. Actisite® maintains a constant concentration in gingival crevicular fluid (GCF) for a period of 10 days, equivalent to 8 μg/mL in systemic intake [65].

Although it has demonstrated clinical benefits [66], Actisite® is no longer used due to its non-biodegradable nature. Moreover, it seems that the application of fibers in periodontal pockets has been associated with a high degree of discomfort for the patient and with inflammatory signs after their removal [2].

Periodontal Plus AB® has emerged as a resorbable variant of tetracycline-impregnated collagen fibers. They are applied in the periodontal pocket and have a resorption period of about 7 days. This system has proven to be effective in terms of probing depth and periodontal clinical attachment loss [67]. Abraham et al. comparatively investigated in an interventional study the effects of additional administration in the periodontal pockets of chlorhexidine gel (Chlo-Site®), metronidazole gel (Metrogyl®) and tetracycline fibers (Periodontal Plus AB®); the authors showed favorable effects on plaque index and gingival index at 30 days for all three methods, but the effects were more significant for tetracycline fibers [68].

9. Semi-solid systems

Semi-solid systems include films, chips or strips that are inserted into the periodontal pocket; the controlled release of the drug is achieved either by its diffusion or by dissolving the carrier system [11]. These devices adapt to the shape and size of the periodontal pocket, are relatively easy to insert and the discomfort felt by patients is minimal [2].

Non-resorbable acrylic systems, with tetracycline or metronidazole as an active substance, were initially investigated [69]; although effective in antibacterial activity, these systems have been shown difficult to manipulate and remove from the periodontal pocket, being also associated with a local inflammatory response [70].

Periochip® is a chip of hydrolyzed gelatin crosslinked with glutaraldehyde, measuring 4.0 × 5.0 × 0.35 μm, containing 2.5 mg of chlorhexidine gluconate [26]. Periochip® releases chlorhexidine in a biphasic manner; in the first 24 hours, about 40% of the drug is released and the rest of the drug is released linearly for 7–10 days [71].

Another similar device is PerioColTM-CG®, which contains approximately 2.5 mg of CHX gluconate in a biodegradable matrix of type 1 collagen derived from freshwater fish [72].

In general, data on the use of these chlorhexidine chips support their effectiveness in reducing periodontal parameters, in association with SRP versus SRP alone, at assessments of 3, 9 and even 12 months postoperatively [73–75].

A number of biodegradable polymers, such as poly-hydroxybutyric acid and poly lactic-co-glycolic acid, atelocollagen, gelatin or chitosan/poly lactic-co-glycolic acid, in the form of tetracycline-impregnated films were investigated with significant reductions of probing depths and inflammation, quantified by bleeding on probing [2]. Moreover, the 25% tetracycline-impregnated polylactic-co-glycolic acid film demonstrated continuous release of the pharmacological agent for 10 days after placement [76].

10. Photodynamic antibacterial therapy

Photodynamic antibacterial therapy (aPDT) is based on the chemical effects of light. The main components involved in photodynamic antibacterial therapy consist of the light energy source, the photosensitizer and molecular oxygen. Their association will generate a flow of reactions with therapeutic effects [77].

Laser radiation can generate a number of bactericidal effects through photothermal effects, even in the absence of a photosensitizing substance. Nd:YAG lasers have selective absorption in pigments, are effective in destroying bacterial species such as *P. gingivalis* [78]. Moreover, laser radiation can decrease the release of bacterial products, such as endotoxins [79]. Thus, photodynamic therapy involves decreasing bacterial activity, inflammatory status, promoting decontamination and healing of affected periodontal sites.

The use of aPDT in adjunctive periodontal therapy can be amplified by applying a photosensitizing substance in the periodontal pocket and irradiating it with a light source (laser or LED) of a wavelength appropriate to the used substance [47, 80]; cytotoxic reactive oxygen species are generated after exposure to light, with effects involving protein, cell membrane and bacterial organ damage [81] (**Figure 2**).

A photosensitizer or photoactivatable agent, such as methylene blue, is applied in the periodontal pocket. Exposure of tissue to light at the appropriate wavelength in the presence of molecular oxygen generates the formation of reactive oxygen species (ROS); ROS causes non-thermal cytotoxic effects by damaging microorganisms' proteins, cell membranes and organelles [47, 82].

Various photosensitizing agents have been investigated in periodontal therapy, including phenothiazine derivatives (methylene blue, toluidine blue), xanthens (erythrosine, eosin-Y, Bengal roses), riboflavin derivatives, indocyanine green, fullerene derivatives, bordipiromethane [47, 83].

Numerous studies have investigated the efficacy of aPDT with methylene blue and toluidine blue, the latter demonstrating higher efficacy. Diode laser and toluidine blue aPDT effects on *Porphyromonas gingivalis* were evaluated [84]; treatment with toluidine blue and 2.2 J/cm^2 light dose reduced *P. gingivalis* by 2.43 log. In another study, black-pigmented bacteria *P. gingivalis* and *P. intermedia* reacted strongly to the 690 nm wavelength toluidine and laser treatment protocol, reducing bacterial growth by up to 2 logs [85].

A research group led by Azizi investigated the efficacy of aPDT with toluidine blue and phenothiazine chloride in the disinfection of zirconium implants contaminated

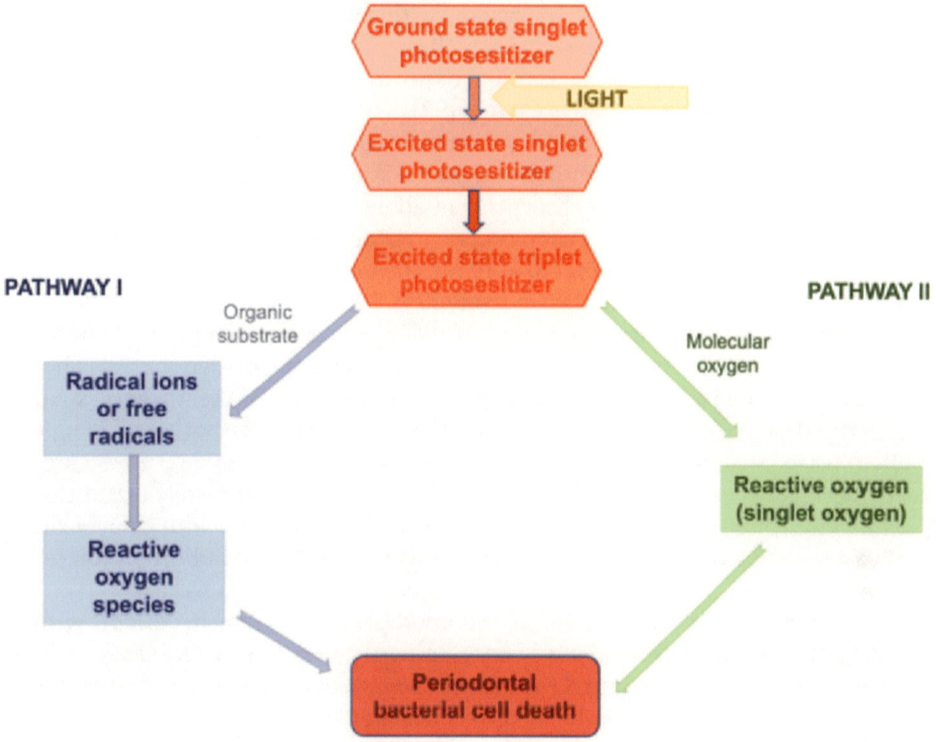

Figure 2.
Mechanism of action in aPDT.

with *P. gingivalis*, *P. intermedia* and *A. actinomycetemcomitans* [86]. Only toluidine blue showed a significant reduction in the number of bacteria; bacterial reductions after aPDT with both photosensitizers were greater than the chlorhexidine positive control.

A strong therapeutic effect has been observed for the association of riboflavin in aPDT against the pathogens *P. gingivalis*, *Fillifactor alocis*, *P. micra*, *Campylobacter rectus*, *Fusobacterium nucleatum*, *Eikenella corrodens* and *P. intermedia* [87].

Indocyanine green has also been evaluated as a potential photosensitizer. It consists of two aromatic parts connected by a polyunsaturated chain; it is a dye commonly used in medicine, especially in imagistic investigations [88]. It penetrates rapidly into tissues and has low toxicity, being approved by the FDA for clinical use and recognized as non-toxic [89].

The absorption range for indocyanine green is between 600 nm and 900 nm and emits fluorescence between 750 nm and 950 nm [90]. Indocyanine green aPDT does not require the presence of oxygen to activate and release free radicals and singlet oxygen [91]; indocyanine green therapy is also called photothermal therapy. Thus, indocyanine green may be more effective than other photosensitizers in the periodontal pocket, an environment characterized by hypoxia. A recent meta-analysis [92] observed statistically significant improvements in aPDT results with indocyanine green at 3 months and 6 months after therapy, compared with single SRP; probing depth demonstrated an average additional reduction of 1.17 mm and 1.06 mm at 3 and 6 months, respectively; for clinical attachment loss, an average additional gain of 0.70 mm and 1.03 mm was observed at 3 and 6 months, respectively [92]. We have recently investigated the effects of 5 mg/mL indocyanine green irradiation by 810 nm diode laser, supplementary to SRP in patients with periodontitis and type II DM, compared to SRP alone. We observed that SRP + aPDT generated more significant reductions in bleeding on probing, probing depth and clinical attachment loss but not for plaque index and HbA1c than SRP alone [93].

Attention has also been paid to the potential of curcumin as a photosensitizing agent. Curcumin absorbs light from the edge of UV and visible radiation, over a range of 300–500 nm, with maximum absorption of about 420 nm [83].

The antibacterial activity of various concentrations of photoactivated turmeric with LED light at a wavelength of 420–480 nm for 1 minute was investigated against *A. actinomycetemcomitans* in an in vitro study [94]. Bacteria with exponential growth were combined with a solution of turmeric concentration ranging from 25 to 0.098 μg/mL; 0.12% chlorhexidine solution was used as a positive control. The results demonstrated a dose-dependent antibacterial activity of the turmeric solution [92]. In the absence of blue light irradiation, the turmeric concentration of 25 μg/mL resulted in a logarithmic reduction of *A. actinomycetemcomitans* of 6.03 ± 0.39 log10; the turmeric concentration of 0.78 μg/mL under irradiation completely eradicated *A. actinomycetemcomitans*, an effect also obtained after co-culture with chlorhexidine 0.12%. At the same time, maximum signal intensity of hydroxyl radical production was observed following the association of turmeric with LED irradiation [47].

Sreedhar et al. observed in a clinical and microbiological study in patients with periodontitis that the additional use of curcumin gel generated an antibacterial effect on *P. gingivalis*, *P. intermedia* and *A. actinomycetemcomitans*, but PDT amplified the benefits of curcumin, further enhanced by repeated PDT sessions [95].

An interesting nano-carrier was designed by Shlar and colleagues who used a curcumin derivative as a photosensitizer; curcumin-loaded cyclodextrin was coated with 5–20 layers of poly-L-lysine, poly-L-glutamic acid and carboxymethyl-β-cyclodextrin (CM-cyclodextrin). CM-cyclodextrin was covalently crosslinked or left unchanged. The authors noted that crosslinking provided greater stability and less release of curcumin [96].

Data in the literature indicate that the bactericidal effects of turmeric as a photosensitizing agent may depend on the type of carrier or solvent used, which may alter the wavelength where the efficiency is maximum [97]. In addition, turmeric has a high rate of photodegradation, which translates into the need to use it almost immediately after preparation [98].

A complex systematic review, conducted by Salvi et al. [99], aimed to investigate the effects of aPDT on SRP in patients with untreated periodontitis after a follow-up of 6 months. The authors observed a high heterogeneity and variability regarding the protocols and the results, with patient-reported benefits still unclear [99].

11. Locally delivered antimicrobials in the current therapeutic guidelines

Based on the current classification system of periodontal conditions [100], and solid findings from randomized controlled trials (RCTs), new guidelines have emerged, providing recommendations for periodontitis treatment stages I-III [101] and IV [102]. According to the proposed guidelines, locally administered sustained-release antimicrobials, such as chlorhexidine (Periochip®) or antibiotics (Atridox®, Arestin®), may be considered as an adjunct to subgingival instrumentation, due to proven efficiency and relatively low risk of side effects [101]. This recommendation is based on a systematic review performed by Herrera et al. [103], which included

50 different studies on locally delivered antimicrobials (gels, chips and fibers); the authors concluded that their use exerted statistically significant benefits in terms of probing depth reduction and short-term clinical attachment gain [103].

Oral rinses with chlorhexidine also might be recommended, for a limited period of time and in specific cases [101], due to its known side effects, and only after optimizing the mechanical plaque control.

With respect to aPDT, the guidelines do not recommend its standard use in periodontitis patients. This decision is based on the high heterogeneity which characterizes the RCTs, with various photosensitizers, laser types, different wavelengths, dosage and number of sessions. Moreover, it is stated that, even if there were no reported adverse effects of aPDT, the high cost of this particular procedure is not justified in standard practice [101].

Drug delivery system	**Active drug**	**Mechanism of delivery**	**Advantages**	**Disadvantages**
Subgingival irrigation	Chlorhexidine Triclosan Antibiotics	Application in the periodontal pocket with the aid of a syringe	Good disease site reaching Adequate concentration in situ Cost saving Easy application	Poor maintenance of drug concentration in time Relatively uncontrolled and inconsistent drug delivery Requires multiple applications Microorganisms' resistance can occur
Gels	Chlorhexidine Tetracycline Metronidazole Doxycycline Minocycline	Application in the periodontal pocket with the aid of a syringe/canula	Patient acceptability Easy application	Poor retention at the site Difficulties in obtaining an accurate dosage
Microparticle systems	Minocycline Ofloxacin	Microspheres in the unit-dose cartridge	Good maintenance of drug concentration in time Can reach even narrow pockets	Resistant microorganisms can emerge
Fibers	Tetracycline HCl Chlorhexidine	Inserted in the periodontal pocket and isolated with the aid of cement	Good maintenance of drug concentration in time	Require a second session for their removal Emergence of resistant microorganisms Signs of local irritation can occur
Films	Chlorhexidine Tetracycline Metronidazole	Flexible polymer inserted in the periodontal pocket	Thin and flexible Easy insertion Less discomfort Prolonged effect High site-specificity	Difficult to apply in narrow, less accessible pockets

Table 1.
Summary of currently available locally delivered antimicrobials.

The indications and the contraindications for the locally delivered antimicrobials are generally the same for all the mentioned systems. They include as follows:
Indications

- Always, as adjunctive to scaling and root planing
- Deep and localized periodontal pockets in patients with periodontitis Grade A or B
- Patients with periodontitis who do not respond to conventional treatment
- Patients with periimplantitis
- Furcation lesions Grade I or II
- Contraindications
- As a replacement for scaling and root planing
- As a replacement for surgical periodontal therapy
- As a replacement for systemic antimicrobial therapy/prophylaxis
- Not a substitute for self-performed plaque control by patients
- Generalized periodontal pockets
- Patients with allergies/contraindications to the specific active drug
- Patients with a history/risk of infective endocarditis, to avoid the risk of bacteriemia

The main advantages and disadvantages of locally delivered antimicrobials are presented in **Table 1**. Additionally, general advantages can be mentioned: drug dosage is lower than for the antibiotics with systemic administration; certain agents cannot be taken through a systemic route (such as chlorhexidine); more adequate local concentration for the active drug.

As general disadvantage, certain techniques might be time-consuming; moreover, due to site-specificity, other bacterial niches from the oral cavity are not reached, including tonsils, buccal mucosa or tongue.

12. Conclusions and future directions

Continuous discoveries in the understanding of the mechanisms which cause periodontal disease, as well as those which accelerate tissue destruction, have led to the development of new methods of treatment. It is clear at this time that non-surgical periodontal debridement by scaling and root planing is often insufficient for the resolution of periodontal disease. Thus, local adjunctive therapy is increasingly used in current practice. Local drug treatment against bacterial plaque, in combination with SRP, involves a wide variety of products already commercially available or under research.

There is currently insufficient data to establish a "gold standard" in local antimicrobial therapy. Current guidelines recommend the usage of oral rinses with chlorhexidine and locally administered sustained-release antimicrobials in the standard treatment of periodontitis patients but in specific cases.

The main concern in the design of these products is to ensure an optimal concentration of the drug in situ and to maintain the long-term potential beneficial effects, without local or systemic complications. Numerous carriers have been investigated over time. In addition to the slow-release products already available, a promising prospect is offered by nanoparticle-based antibacterial therapy or aPDT therapy.

Moreover, the current research directions are focused on the development of multi-component products, with the incorporation of agents to produce not only the disinfection of periodontal pockets but also a resolution of inflammation at the molecular level.

Of course, SRP remains a *sine qua non* condition in periodontal therapy for the disorganization of bacterial biofilm, but current trends suggest a much more complex therapeutic intervention, individualized per patient, with complex and complete addressing of the factors which maintain and aggravate the periodontal disease. In our opinion, the identification of a universally effective adjunctive therapy product is a utopia precisely because of the variability of periodontal disease etiopathogenesis. We believe that it is crucial not only to know the available products but also to identify the most effective compound and technique for the patient in the dental chair.

Author details

Irina-Georgeta Sufaru[1*], Maria-Alexandra Martu[1], Ionut Luchian[1], Silvia Teslaru[1], Simona Stoleriu[1], Stefan-Ioan Stratul[2], Darian Rusu[2], Monica Silvia Tatarciuc[1] and Sorina Mihaela Solomon[1]

1 Faculty of Dental Medicine, Grigore T. Popa University of Medicine and Pharmacy Iasi, Romania

2 Anton Sculean Center for Research of Periodontal and Peri-implant Diseases, Victor Babes University of Medicine and Pharmacy Timisoara, Romania

*Address all correspondence to: irina_ursarescu@yahoo.com

References

[1] Meyle J, Chapple I. Molecular aspects of the pathogenesis of periodontitis. Periodontology 2000. 2015;**69**:7-17. DOI: 10.1111/prd.12104

[2] Wei Y, Deng Y, Ma S, Ran M, Jia Y, Meng J, et al. Local drug delivery systems as therapeutic strategies against periodontitis: A systematic review. Journal of Controlled Release. 2021;**333**:269-282. DOI: 10.1016/j.jconrel.2021.03.041

[3] Tonetti MS, Greenwell H, Kornman KS. Staging and grading of periodontitis: Framework and proposal of a new classification and case definition. Journal of Periodontology. 2018;**89**:S159-S172. DOI: 10.1002/JPER.18-0006

[4] Lopez R, Hujoel P, Belibasakis N. On putative periodontal pathogens: An epidemiological perspective. Virulence. 2015;**6**:249-257. DOI: 10.1080/21505594.2015.1014266

[5] Van Dyke TE, Bartold PM, Reynolds EC. The nexus between periodontal inflammation and dysbiosis. Frontiers in Immunology. 2020;**11**:511. DOI: 10.3389/fimmu.2020.00511

[6] Lim G, Janu U, Chiou LL, Gandhi KK, Palomo L, John V. Periodontal health and systemic conditions. Dentistry Journal. 2020;**8**:130. DOI: 10.3390/dj8040130

[7] Germen M, Baser U, Lacin CC, Firath E, Issever H, Yalcin F. Periodontitis prevalence, severity, and risk factors: A comparison of the AAP/CDC case definition and the EFP/AAP classification. International Journal of Environmental Research and Public Health. 2021;**18**:3459. DOI: 10.3390/ijerph18073459

[8] Mann J, Bernstein Y, Findler M. Periodontal disease and its prevention, by traditional and new avenues (review). Experimental and Therapeutic Medicine. 2020;**19**:1504-1506. DOI: 10.3892/etm.2019.8381

[9] Addy M, Martin MV. Systemic antimicrobials in the treatment of chronic periodontal diseases: A dilemma. Oral Diseases. 2003;**9**:38-44. DOI: 10.1034/j.1601-0825.9.s1.7.x

[10] Jain KK. Current status and future prospects of drug delivery systems. Methods in Molecular Biology. 2014;**1141**: 1-56. DOI: 10.1007/978-1-4939-0363-4_1

[11] Sholapurkar A, Sharma D, Glass B, Miller C, Nimmo A, Jennings E. Professionally delivered local antimicrobials in the treatment of patients with periodontitis—A narrative review. Dental Journal. 2021;**9**:2. DOI: 10.3390/dj9010002

[12] Rajeshwari HR, Dhamecha D, Jagwani S, Rao M, Jadhav K, Shaikh S, et al. Local drug delivery systems in the management of periodontitis: A scientific review. Journal of Controlled Release. 2019;**307**:393-409. DOI: 10.1016/j.jconrel.2019.06.038

[13] Daudt FA, Rösing CK, Chiapinotto GA, Oppermann RV. Effect of the topical application of triclosan in periodontally treated patients. Acta Odontológica Latinoamericana. 2011;**24**:205-210

[14] Galván M, Gonzalez S, Cohen CL, Alonaizan FA, Chen CTL, Rich SK, et al. Periodontal effects of 0.25% sodium hypochlorite twice-weekly oral rinse. A pilot study. Journal of Periodontal Research. 2013;**49**:696-702. DOI: 10.1111/jre.12151

[15] Al Habashneh R, Alsalman W, Khader Y. Ozone as an adjunct to conventional nonsurgical therapy in chronic periodontitis: A randomized controlled clinical trial. Journal of Periodontal Research. 2015;**50**:37-43. DOI: 10.1111/jre.12177

[16] Sindhura H, Harsha RH, Shilpa RH. Efficacy of subgingival irrigation with 10% povidone-iodine as an adjunct to scaling and root planing: A clinical and microbiological study. Indian Journal of Dental Research. 2017;**28**:514-518. DOI: 10.4103/ijdr.IJDR_497_15

[17] Hallmon WW, Rees TD. Local anti-infective therapy: Mechanical and physical approaches. A systematic review. Annals of Periodontology. 2003;**8**:99-114. DOI: 10.1902/annals.2003.8.1.99

[18] Hanes PJ, Purvis JP. Local anti-infective therapy: Pharmacological agents. A systematic review. Annals of Periodontology. 2003;**8**:79-98. DOI: 10.1902/annals.2003.8.1.79

[19] Sahrmann P, Puhan MA, Attin T, Schmidlin PR. Systematic review on the effect of rinsing with povidone-iodine during nonsurgical periodontal therapy. Journal of Periodontal Research. 2010;**45**:153-164. DOI: 10.1111/j.1600-0765.2009.01232.x

[20] Bizzarro S, Vander Velden U, Loos BG. Local disinfection with sodium hypochlorite as adjunct to basic periodontal therapy: A randomized controlled trial. Journal of Clinical Periodontology. 2016;**43**:778-788. DOI: 10.1111/jcpe.12578

[21] da Costa L, Amaral C, Barbirato DDS, Leao ATT, Fogacci MF. Chlorhexidine mouthwash as an adjunct to mechanical therapy in chronic periodontitis: A meta-analysis. Journal of the American Dental Association. 2017;**148**:308-318. DOI: 10.1016/j.adaj.2017.01.021

[22] Isola G, Polizzi A, Santonocito S, Dalessandri D, Migliorati M, Indelicato F. New frontiers on adjuvants drug strategies and treatments in periodontitis. Scientia Pharmaceutica. 2021;**89**:46. DOI: 10.3390/scipharm89040046

[23] Bracke J, Basara M, Savord E, Dunaway A, Watkins M. Pilot evaluation of a simple adjunctive method for improved removal of oral biofilm during conventional scaling and root planing therapy. Journal of Biological Regulators and Homeostatic Agents. 2015;**29**:6-9

[24] Isola G, Matarese G, Williams RC, Siciliano VI, Alibrandi A, Cordasco G, et al. The effects of a desiccant agent in the treatment of chronic periodontitis: A randomized, controlled clinical trial. Clinical Oral Investigations. 2018;**22**:791-800. DOI: 10.1007/s00784-017-2154-7

[25] Sufaru IG, Lazar L, Sincar DC, Martu MA, Pasarin L, Luca EO, et al. Clinical effects of locally delivered lactobacillus reuteri as adjunctive therapy in patients with periodontitis: A split-mouth study. Applied Sciences. 2022;**12**:2470. DOI: 10.3390/app12052470

[26] Tan OI, Safii SH, Razali M. Commercial local pharmacotherapeutics and adjunctive agents for nonsurgical treatment of periodontitis: A contemporary review of clinical efficacies and challenges. Antibiotics. 2019;**9**:11. DOI: 10.3390/antibiotics9010011

[27] Cosyn J, Wyn I, De Rouck T, Sabzevar MM. Long-term clinical effects of a chlorhexidine varnish implemented treatment strategy for chronic periodontitis. Journal of Periodontology. 2006;**77**:406-415. DOI: 10.1902/jop.2006.050144

[28] Manthena S, Ramesh A, Srikanth A, Ramoji Rao MV, Preethi PL, Samatha YP. Comparative evaluation of subgingivally delivered chlorhexidine varnish and chlorhexidine gel in reducing microbial count after mechanical periodontal therapy. Journal of Basic and Clinical Pharmacy. 2015;**6**:24-28. DOI: 10.4103/0976-0105.145775

[29] Manikandan D, Balaji VR, Niazi TM, Rohini G, Karthikeyan B, Jesudoss P. Chlorhexidine varnish implemented treatment strategy for chronic periodontitis: A clinical and microbial study. Journal of Pharmacy & Bioallied Sciences. 2016;**8**:S133-S137. DOI: 10.4103/0975-7406.191943

[30] Sachdeva S, Grover V, Malhotra R, Kapoor A, Mohanty K. Comparison of clinical effectiveness of single and multiple applications of 1% chlorhexidine varnish (Cervitec plus) along with scaling and root planing in patients with chronic periodontitis. Journal of Indian Society of Periodontology. 2018;**22**:523-528. DOI: 10.4103/jisp.jisp_252_18

[31] Jain M, Dave D, Jain P, Manohar B, Yadav B, Shetty N. Efficacy of xanthan based chlorhexidine gel as an adjunct to scaling and root planing in treatment of the chronic periodontitis. Journal of Indian Society of Periodontology. 2013;**17**:439-443. DOI: 10.4103/0972-124X.118313

[32] Shamami MS, Faramarzi M, Shirmohmmadi A, Chitsazi M, Ghanitab S. The clinical and metabolic effects of subgingival application of xanthan-based chlorhexidine gel in type 2 diabetic patients with chronic periodontitis. Dental Research Journal. 2016;**14**:299-305. DOI: 10.4103/1735-3327.215961

[33] Stoller NH, Johnson LR, Trapnell S, Harrold CQ, Garrett S. The pharmacokinetic profile of a biodegradable controlled-release delivery system containing doxycycline compared to systemically delivered doxycycline in gingival crevicular fluid, saliva, and serum. Journal of Periodontology. 1998;**69**:1085-1091. DOI: 10.1902/jop.1998.69.10.1085

[34] Ahamed S, Jalaluddin M, Khalid I, Moon N, Shaf TK, Ali FM. The use of controlled release locally delivered 10% doxycycline hyclate gel as an adjunct to scaling and root planing in the treatment of chronic periodontitis: Clinical and microbiological results. The Journal of Contemporary Dental Practice. 2013;**14**:1080-1086. DOI: 10.5005/jp-journals-10024-1455

[35] Tonetti MS, Lang NP, Cortellini P, Suvan JE, Eickholz P, Fourmousis I, et al. Effects of a single topical doxycycline administration adjunctive to mechanical debridement in patients with persistent/recurrent periodontitis but acceptable oral hygiene during supportive periodontal therapy. Journal of Clinical Periodontology. 2012;**39**:475-482. DOI: 10.1111/j.1600-051X.2012.01864.x

[36] Garrett S, Johnson L, Drisko CH, et al. Two multi-center studies evaluating locally delivered doxycycline hyclate, placebo control, oral hygiene, and scaling and root planing in the treatment of periodontitis. Journal of Periodontology. 1999;**70**:490-503. DOI: 10.1902/jop.1999.70.5.490

[37] van Steenberghe D, Bercy P, Kohl J, et al. Subgingival minocycline hydrochloride ointment in moderate to severe chronic adult periodontitis: A randomized, double-blind, vehicle-controlled, multicenter study. Journal of Periodontology. 1993;**64**:637-644. DOI: 10.1902/jop.1993.64.7.637

[38] Wang X, Ma J, Zhu X, Wang F, Zhou L. Minocycline-loaded in situ

hydrogel for periodontitis treatment. Current Drug Delivery. 2018;**15**:664-671. DOI: 10.2174/1567201814666171120120421

[39] Norling T, Lading P, Engström S, Larsson K, Krog N, Nissen SS. Formulation of a drug delivery system based on a mixture of monoglycerides and triglycerides for use in the treatment of periodontal disease. Journal of Clinical Periodontology. 1992;**19**:687-692. DOI: 10.1111/j.1600-051x.1992.tb02529.x

[40] Stoltze K, Stellfeld M. Systemic absorption of metronidazole after application of a metronidazole 25% dental gel. Journal of Clinical Periodontology. 1992;**19**:693-697

[41] Miani PK, do Nascimento C, Sato S, Filho AV, da Fonseca MJ, Pedrazzi V. In vivo evaluation of a metronidazole-containing gel for the adjuvant treatment of chronic periodontitis: Preliminary results. European Journal of Clinical Microbiology & Infectious Diseases. 2011;**31**:1611-1618. DOI: 10.1007/s10096-011-1484-7

[42] Vaish S, Dodwad V, Tyagi P. Clinical efficacy of subgingivally delivered 0.5% controlled release azithromycin gel in the management of chronic periodontitis. Indian Journal of Medical Sciences. 2011;**65**:223-230

[43] Flemming TF, Petersilka G, Völp A, Gravemeier M, Zilly M, Mross D, et al. Efficacy and safety of adjunctive local moxifloxacin delivery in the treatment of periodontitis. Journal of Periodontology. 2011;**82**:96-105. DOI: 10.1902/jop.2010.100124

[44] Priyanka N, Kalra N, Saquib S, Malgaonkar N, Tarakji B, Varsha J, et al. Efficacy of subgingivally delivered satranidazole in the treatment of type 2 diabetes subjects with chronic periodontitis: A randomized controlled clinical trial. Journal of the International Academy of Periodontology. 2015;**17**:42-48

[45] Nakajima M, Tanner EEL, Nakajima N, Ibsen KN, Mitragotri S. Topical treatment of periodontitis using an iongel. Biomaterials. 2021;**276**:121069

[46] Debnath K, Chatterjee A, Priya V. Evaluation of Nano-BioFusion gel as an adjunct to scaling and root planing in chronic periodontitis: A clinico-microbiological study. Journal of Indian Society of Periodontology. 2016;**20**:543. DOI: 10.4103/0972-124X.201696

[47] Solomon SM, Stafie CS, Sufaru IG, Teslaru S, Ghiciuc CM, Petrariu FD, et al. Curcumin as a natural approach of periodontal adjunctive treatment and its immunological implications: A narrative review. Pharmaceutics. 2022;**14**:982. DOI: 10.3390/pharmaceutics14050982

[48] Dave DH, Patel P, Shah M, Dadawala SM, Saraiya K, Sant AV. Comparative evaluation of efficacy of oral curcumin gel as an adjunct to scaling and root planing in the treatment of chronic periodontitis. Advances in Human Biology. 2019;**8**:79-82. DOI: 10.4103/AIHB.AIHB_46_17

[49] Kandwal A, Mamgain RK, Mamgain P. Comparative evaluation of turmeric gel with 2% chlorhexidine gluconate gel for treatment of plaque induced gingivitis: A randomized controlled clinical trial. Ayu. 2015;**36**:145-150. DOI: 10.4103/0974-8520.175537

[50] Bhatia M, Urolagin SS, Pentyala KB, Urolagin SB, Bhoi S. Novel therapeutic approach for the treatment of periodontitis by curcumin. Journal of Clinical and Diagnostic Research. 2014;**8**:ZC65-ZC69. DOI: 10.7860/JCDR/2014/8231.5343

[51] Nasra MM, Khiri HM, Hazzah HA, Abdallah OY. Formulation, in-vitro characterization and clinical evaluation of curcumin in-situ gel for treatment of periodontitis. Drug Delivery. 2017;**24**:133-142. DOI: 10.1080/10717544.2016.1233591

[52] Williams RC, Paquette DW, Offenbacher S, et al. Treatment of periodontitis by local administration of minocycline microspheres: A controlled trial. Journal of Periodontology. 2001;**72**:1535-1544. DOI: 10.1902/jop.2001.72.11.1535

[53] Srirangarajan S, Mundargi RC, Ravindra S, Setty SB, Aminabhavi TM, Thakur S. Randomized, controlled, single-masked, clinical study to compare and evaluate the efficacy of microspheres and gel in periodontal pocket therapy. Journal of Periodontology. 2011;**82**:114-121. DOI: 10.1902/jop.2010.100324

[54] Chiappe VB, Gómez MV, Rodríguez C, Fresolone M, Romanelli HJ. Subgingivally applied minocycline microgranules in subjects with chronic periodontitis: A randomized clinical and microbiological trial. Acta Odontológica Latinoamericana. 2015;**28**:122-131. DOI: 10.1590/S1852-48342015000200005

[55] Laza GM, Sufaru IG, Martu MA, Martu C, Diaconu-Popa DA, Jelihovschi I, et al. Effects of locally delivered minocycline microspheres in postmenopausal female patients with periodontitis: A clinical and microbiological study. Diagnostics. 2022;**12**:1310. DOI: 10.3390/diagnostics12061310

[56] Moura LA, Ribeiro FV, Aiello TB, Duek EA, Sallum EA, Nociti Junior FH, et al. Characterization of the release profile of doxycycline by PLGA microspheres adjunct to non-surgical periodontal therapy. Journal of Biomaterials Science. Polymer Edition. 2015;**26**:573-584. DOI: 10.1080/09205063.2015.1045249

[57] Ali M, Walboomers F, Jansen JA, Yang F. Influence of formulation parameters on encapsulation of doxycycline in PLGA microspheres prepared by double emulsion technique for the treatment of periodontitis. Journal of Drug Delivery Science and Technology. 2019;**52**:263-271. DOI: 10.1016/j.jddst.2019.04.031

[58] Gad HA, Kamel AO, Ezzat OM, El Dessouky HF, Sammour OA. Doxycycline hydrochloride-metronidazole solid lipid microparticles gels for treatment of periodontitis: Development, in-vitro and in-vivo clinical evaluation. Expert Opinion on Drug Delivery. 2017;**14**:1241-1251. DOI: 10.1080/17425247.2017.1329297

[59] Wang TB, Wang J, Shao J, Kouwer PHJ, Bronkhorst EM. A tunable and injectable local drug delivery system for personalized periodontal application. Journal of Controlled Release. 2020;**324**:134-145. DOI: 10.1016/j.jconrel.2020.05.004

[60] Killicarslan M, Gumustas M, Yildiz S, Baykara T. Preparation and characterization of chitosan-based spray-dried microparticles for the delivery of clindamycin phosphate to periodontal pockets. Current Drug Delivery. 2014;**11**:98-111. DOI: 10.2174/15672018113109990055

[61] Yao W, Xu P, Pang Z, Zhao J, Chai Z, Li X, et al. Local delivery of minocycline-loaded PEG-PLA nanoparticles for the enhanced treatment of periodontitis in dogs. International Journal of Nanomedicine. 2014;**9**:3963-3970. DOI: 10.2147/IJN.S67521

[62] Xu S, Zhou Q, Jiang Z, Wang Y, Yang K, Qiu X, et al. The effect of doxycycline-containing chitosan/

carboxymethyl chitosan nanoparticles on NLRP3 inflammasome in periodontal disease. Carbohydrate Polymers. 2020;**237**:116163. DOI: 10.1016/j.carbpol.2020.116163

[63] Joshi D, Garg T, Goyal AK, Rath G. Advanced drug delivery approaches against periodontitis. Drug Delivery. 2016;**23**:363-377. DOI: 10.3109/10717544.2014.935531

[64] Liu D, Yang PS. Minocycline hydrochloride nanoliposomes inhibit the production of TNF-a in LPS-stimulated macrophages. International Journal of Nanomedicine. 2012;**7**:4769-4775. DOI: 10.2147/IJN.S34036

[65] Tonetti M, Cugini MA, Goodson JM. Zero-order delivery with periodontal placement of tetracycline- loaded ethylene vinyl acetate fibers. Journal of Periodontal Research. 1990;**25**:243-249. DOI: 10.1111/j.1600-0765.1990.tb00911.x

[66] Litch JM, Encarnacion M, Chen S, Leonard J, Burkoth TL. Use of the polymeric matrix as internal standard for quantitation of in vivo delivery of tetracycline HCl from Actisite tetracycline fiber during periodontal treatment. Journal of Periodontal Research. 1996;**31**:540-544. DOI: 10.1111/j.1600-0765.1996.tb00518.x

[67] Khan FY, Jan SM, Mushtaq M. Clinical utility of locally-delivered collagen-based biodegradable tetracycline fibers in periodontal therapy: An in vivo study. Journal of Investigative and Clinical Dentistry. 2014;**6**:307-312. DOI: 10.1111/jicd.12111

[68] Abraham A, Raghavan R, Joseph A, Shyamala Devi MP, Varghese M, Sreedevi. Evaluation of different local drug delivery systems in the management of chronic periodontitis: A comparative study. The Journal of Contemporary Dental Practice. 2020;**21**:280-284

[69] Deasy PB, Collins AE, MacCarthy DJ, Russell RJ. Use of strips containing tetracycline hydrochloride or metronidazole for the treatment of advanced periodontal disease. The Journal of Pharmacy and Pharmacology. 1989;**41**:694-699. DOI: 10.1111/j.2042-7158.1989.tb06343.x

[70] Larsen T. In vitro release of doxycycline from bioabsorbable materials and acrylic strips. Journal of Periodontology. 1990;**61**:30-34. DOI: 10.1902/jop.1990.61.1.30

[71] Soskolne WA, Chajek T, Flashner M, Landau I, Stabholtz A, Kolatch B, et al. An in vivo study of the chlorhexidine release profile of the PerioChip in the gingival crevicular fluid, plasma and urine. Journal of Clinical Periodontology. 1998;**25**:1017-1021. DOI: 10.1111/j.1600-051x.1998.tb02407.x

[72] John P, Lazarus F, George JP, Selvam A, Prabhuji MLV. Adjunctive effects of a piscean collagen-based controlled-release chlorhexidine chip in the treatment of chronic periodontitis: A clinical and microbiological study. Journal of Clinical and Diagnostic Research. 2015;**9**:ZC70-ZC74. DOI: 10.7860/JCDR/2015/11534.5965

[73] Carvalho J, Novak MJ, Mota LF. Evaluation of effect of subgingival placement of chlorhexidine chips as an adjunct to scaling and root planing. Journal of Periodontology. 2007;**78**:997-1001. DOI: 10.1902/jop.2007.060122

[74] Reddy BVR, Chava VK, Kumar AJ. Effect of chlorhexidine chip in the treatment of chronic periodontitis. Journal of Natural Science, Biology, and Medicine. 2014;**5**:268-272. DOI: 10.4103/0976-9668.136159

[75] Konuganti K, Kumar A. Efficacy of subgingivally delivered flurbiprofen and chlorhexidine chip in the treatment of chronic periodontitis—A randomized controlled clinical trial. International Journal of Pharmaceutical Sciences Review and Research. 2016;**40**:149-153

[76] Maze GI, Reinhardt RA, Agarwal RK, Dyer JK, Robinson DH, DuBois LM, et al. Response to intracrevicular controlled delivery of 25% tetracycline from poly(lactide/glycolide) film strips in SPT patients. Journal of Clinical Periodontology. 1995;**22**:860-867. DOI: 10.1111/j.1600-051x.1995.tb01785.x

[77] Chilakamarthi U, Giribabu L. Photodynamic therapy: Past, present and future. Chemical Record. 2017;**17**:775-802. DOI: 10.1002/tcr.201600121

[78] Akiyama F, Aoki A, Miura-Uchiyama M, Sasaki KM, Ichinose S, Umeda M, et al. In vitro studies of the ablation mechanism of periodontopathic bacteria and decontamination effect on periodontally diseased root surfaces by erbium:Yttrium-aluminum-garnet laser. Lasers in Medical Science. 2011;**26**:193-204. DOI: 10.1007/s10103-010-0763-3

[79] Folwaczny M, Aggstaller H, Mehl A, Hickel R. Removal of bacterial endotoxin from root surface with Er:YAG laser. American Journal of Dentistry. 2003;**16**:3-5

[80] Dobson J, de Queiroz GF, Golding JP. Photodynamic therapy and diagnosis: Principles and comparative aspects. Veterinary Journal. 2018;**233**:8-18. DOI: 10.1016/j.tvjl.2017.11.012

[81] Jori G, Fabris C, Soncin M, Ferro S, Coppellotti O, Dei D, et al. Photodynamic therapy in the treatment of microbial infections: Basic principles and perspective applications. Lasers in Surgery and Medicine. 2006;**38**:468-481. DOI: 10.1002/lsm.20361

[82] Meisel P, Kocher T. Photodynamic therapy for periodontal diseases: State of the art. Journal of Photochemistry and Photobiology B: Biology. 2005;**79**:159-170. DOI: 10.1016/j.jphotobiol.2004.11.023

[83] Sobotta L, Skupin-Mrugalska P, Piskorz J, Mielcarek J. Non-porphyrinoid photosensitizers mediated photodynamic inactivation against bacteria. Dyes and Pigments. 2019;**163**:337-355. DOI: 10.1016/j.ejmech.2019.04.057

[84] Matevski D, Weersink R, Tenenbaum HC, Wilson B, Ellen RP, Lépine G. Lethal photosensitization of periodontal pathogens by a red-filtered xenon lamp in vitro. Journal of Periodontal Research. 2003;**38**:428-435. DOI: 10.1034/j.1600-0765.2003.00673.x

[85] Dörtbudak O, Haas R, Bernhart T, Mailath-Pokorny G. Lethal photosensitization for decontamination of implant surfaces in the treatment of peri-implantitis. Clinical Oral Implants Research. 2001;**12**:104-108. DOI: 10.1034/j.1600-0501.2001.012002104.x

[86] Azizi B, Budimir A, Bago I, et al. Antimicrobial efficacy of photodynamic therapy and light-activated disinfection on contaminated zirconia implants: An in vitro study. Photodiagnosis and Photodynamic Therapy. 2018;**21**:328-333. DOI: 10.1016/j.pdpdt.2018.01.017

[87] Nielsen HK, Garcia J, Væth M, Schlafer S. Comparison of riboflavin and toluidine blue O as photosensitizers for photoactivated disinfection on endodontic and periodontal pathogens in vitro. PLoS One. 2015;**10**:e0140720. DOI: 10.1371/journal.pone.0140720

[88] Qi S, Zhang H, Wang X, Lv J, Liu D, Shen W, et al. Development of a NIR fluorescent probe for highly selective

and sensitive detection of cysteine in living cells and in vivo. Talanta. 2021;**234**:122685. DOI: 10.1016/j.talanta.2021.122685

[89] Porcu EP, Salis A, Gavini E, Rassu G, Maestri M, Giunchedi P. Indocyanine green delivery systems for tumour detection and treatments. Biotechnology Advances. 2016;**34**:768-789. DOI: 10.1016/j.biotechadv.2016.04.001

[90] Houthoofd S, Vuylsteke M, Mordon S, Fourneau I. Photodynamic therapy for atherosclerosis. The potential of indocyanine green. Photodiagnosis and Photodynamic Therapy. 2020;**29**:101568. DOI: 10.1016/j.pdpdt.2019.10.003

[91] Yoon HJ, Lee HS, Lim JY, Park JH. Liposomal indocyanine green for enhanced photothermal therapy. ACS Applied Materials & Interfaces. 2017;**9**:5683-5691

[92] Bashir NZ, Singh HA, Virdee SS. Indocyanine green–mediated antimicrobial photodynamic therapy as an adjunct to periodontal therapy: A systematic review and meta-analysis. Clinical Oral Investigations. 2021;**25**:5699-5710. DOI: 10.1007/s00784-021-03871-2

[93] Sufaru IG, Martu MA, Luchian I, Stoleriu S, Diaconu-Popa D, Martu C, et al. The effects of 810 nm diode laser and indocyanine green on periodontal parameters and HbA1c in patients with periodontitis and type II diabetes mellitus: A randomized controlled study. Diagnostics. 2022;**12**:1614. DOI: 10.3390/diagnostics12071614

[94] Saitawee D, Teerakapong A, Morales NP, Jitprasertwong P, Hormdee D. Photodynamic therapy of Curcuma longa extract stimulated with blue light against Aggregatibacter actinomycetemcomitans. Photodiagnosis and Photodynamic Therapy. 2018;**22**:101-105. DOI: 10.1016/j.pdpdt.2018.03.001

[95] Sreedhar A, Sarkar I, Rajan P, Pai J, Malagi S, Kamath V, et al. Comparative evaluation of the efficacy of curcumin gel with and without photo activation as an adjunct to scaling and root planing in the treatment of chronic periodontitis: A split mouth clinical and microbiological study. Journal of Natural Science, Biology, and Medicine. 2015;**6**:S102-S109. DOI: 10.4103/0976-9668.166100

[96] Shlar I, Droby S, Rodov V. Antimicrobial coatings on polyethylene terephthalate based on curcumin/cyclodextrin complex embedded in a multilayer polyelectrolyte architecture. Colloids and Surfaces. B, Biointerfaces. 2018;**164**:379-387. DOI: 10.1016/j.colsurfb.2018.02.008

[97] Dovigo LN, Carmello JC, Costa CAS, Vergani CE, Brunetti IL, Bagnato VS, et al. Curcumin-mediated photodynamic inactivation of Candida albicans in a murine model of oral candidiasis. Medical Mycology. 2013;**51**:243-251. DOI: 10.3109/13693786.2012.714081

[98] Hegge AB, Vukicevic M, Bruzell E, Kristensen S, Tønnesen HH. Solid dispersions for preparation of phototoxic supersaturated solutions for antimicrobial photodynamic therapy (aPDT) studies on curcumin and curcuminoides L. European Journal of Pharmaceutics and Biopharmaceutics. 2013;**83**:95-105. DOI: 10.1016/j.ejpb.2012.09.011

[99] Salvi GE, Stahl A, Schmidt JC, Ramseier CA, Sculean A, Walter C. Adjunctive laser or antimicrobial photodynamic therapy to non-surgical mechanical instrumentation in patients with untreated periodontitis. A systematic review and meta-analysis.

Journal of Clinical Periodontology. 2020;**47**:176-198. DOI: 10.1111/jcpe.13236

[100] Caton JG, Armitage G, Beglundh T, Chapple ILC, Jepsen S, Kornman KS, et al. A new classification scheme for periodontal and peri-implant diseases and conditions—Introduction and key changes from the 1999 classification. Journal of Clinical Periodontology. 2018;**45**:S1-S8. DOI: 10.1111/jcpe.12935

[101] Sanz M, Herrera D, Kebschull M, Chapple I, Jepsen S, Beglundh T, et al. Treatment of stage I-III periodontitis—The EFP S3 level clinical practice guideline. Journal of Clinical Periodontology. 2020;**47**:4-60. DOI: 10.1111/jcpe.13290

[102] Herrera D, Sanz M, Kebschull M, Jepsen S, Sculean A, Beglundh T, et al. Treatment of stage IV periodontitis—The EFP S3 level clinical practice guideline. Journal of Clinical Periodontology. 2022;**49**:4-71. DOI: 10.1111/jcpe.13639

[103] Herrera D, Matesanz P, Martin C, Oud V, Feres M, Teughels W. Adjunctive effect of locally delivered antimicrobials in periodontitis therapy: A systematic review and meta-analysis. Journal of Clinical Periodontology. 2020;**47**: 239-256. DOI: 10.1111/jcpe.13230

Chapter 9

Trans-Resveratrol: From Phytonutrient Supplement, to Novel Nanotherapeutic Agent

Tracey Lynn Harney

Abstract

Trans-resveratrol (3,5,4′-trihydroxy-trans-stilbene) (RES) is a plant polyphenol that has been well documented for its anti-oxidant, antimicrobial, anti-inflammatory, and anti-aging properties. Moreover, compelling evidence presented in the abundance of pre-clinical studies using ligature-induced periodontitis models has positioned RES as a theoretically viable candidate for the reduction of the chronic inflammation, oxidative stress, and tissue destruction seen in periodontitis (PD). However, the instability of RES under physiological conditions, as well as its rapid hepatic clearance, has presented as a challenge to its ubiquitous application as an oral therapeutic in clinical practice. Fortunately, with the application of nanotechnology, the pharmacological profile of RES repositions the phytochemical from an herb-based supplement, useful as an adjunct therapy, to a stable and potent nanomedicine, demonstrating efficacy for the prevention and treatment of PD and its associated systemic diseases. This chapter explores the details of the potential for nano-RES as a viable therapeutic for PD.

Keywords: periodontitis, polyphenols, trans-resveratrol (RES), pharmacognosy, nanotechnology

1. Introduction

Periodontal Disease (PD) is a complex and multifactorial chronic systemic inflammatory condition that manifests via the interplay between dysbiosis of the normal microbiota of the oral cavity, and the dysregulation of the host immune response [1] The shift in the microbiota toward pathogenic organisms, activates host inflammation which persists if left untreated, ultimately progressing to continuous tissue destruction of the supporting tissues around the tooth. The clinical manifestations that result are bleeding gums, gradual tooth detachment and bone loss, which can be painful, and potentially result in edentulism, if left unchecked [1].

Since the global prevalence of PD of some form, is positioned at approximately 50% of the adult population, the growing concern around this approximation is particularly necessary, when one reflects upon the extensive list of immune-related systemic diseases with which PD is associated [2–4]. That is, PD has been associated with cardiovascular [5–11], gastrointestinal, respiratory, renal, hepatic, neurodegenerative, and autoimmune disease; obesity, diabetes, viral infections, adverse pregnancy outcomes and some cancers have also been reported to be associated with PD. Moreover, due to the systemic nature of immune dysregulation and pathogenic dysbiosis, the relationship between PD and many of these comorbidities is bidirectional [12].

One cannot emphasize more, the multifaceted pathogenesis of PD, which involves the interchange between the host tissues and the accompanying microbial communities of the oral cavity, and the microenvironment therein. For this reason, clarification of the details of the pathogenic mechanisms continues to unfold. Fortunately, knowledge gained from studies on the oral microbiome, has recently emerged [13–15].

In this way, understanding further details of the disease process of PD from the perspective of the oral microbiome can assist in the creation of novel preventative and therapeutic applications.

The oral microbiome (OM), which has been estimated to consist of greater than 10^8 microbes per milliliter of saliva, is considered by many, as one of the most clinically important collections of microbial organisms in the human body [16]. Both prokaryotic and eukaryotic microorganisms make up the estimated 1000 microbial species of the OM. However, more than 700 microbes are prokaryotic, giving investigators a rationale for focusing on the bacterial taxa of the oral cavity when seeking to answer questions about the nature of oral health and disease [17–19].

Practicably, by gaining a deeper understanding of the mechanisms employed by "keystone" bacterial essential players, which are Gram negative anaerobes (e.g., red-complex pathogens, *Porphyromonas gingivalis (Pg)*, *Treponema denticola* and *Tannerella forsythia*) in the inflammation process, one may be in a better position to produce an effective and up-to-date arsenal of remedies for the prevention, management, and resolution of PD [20].

It is worth noting that part of the survival mechanism for Gram negative bacteria is the dissemination of outer membrane vesicles containing various virulence factors which result in a distorted immunological dysregulation and tissue destruction [21, 22]. This strategy is a likely explanation for the discovery of pathogenic bacterial DNA at sites distal from the oral cavity. Further to this, Gram negative bacteria contain the virulence factor lipopolysaccharide (LPS) in their outer membrane, which acts as a constant inflammatory trigger via its pathogen-associated molecular patterning (PAMP). Interestingly, antibiotic therapy is not a straight forward solution, since dead Gram negatives also release LPS [23].

The treatment principle of PD is founded in the elimination of the pathogenic dysbiotic biofilm, whilst addressing the dysregulated immune response of the host. These treatment goals are first addressed via the mechanical removal of subgingival pathogenic dysbiotic plaque and tartar buildup, which is accomplished by the gold standard procedure, scaling and root planning (SRP). As a general rule, SRP is followed by lifelong comprehensive care, which may include subgingival irrigation with antibiotic solutions (www.NHS.uk; www.ADA.org). However, instances involving extensive tissue destruction require surgical intervention, which is more invasive and can be costly. Additionally, as a supplementary treatment, host modulation therapy (HMT) may be employed to address the dysregulation of the immune system that was triggered by dysbiosis [24].

Some phytochemicals have been identified as potential modulators of dysbiotic oral biofilms as well as mitigators of host inflammatory responses (e.g., Curcumin, Hesperidin, Silymarin, Resveratrol) [25–27]. Pharmacognosy, therefore, has been explored as a contributing modality for the mitigation of inflammatory disease.

Indeed, there is a body of evidence in the scientific literature outlining the potential of various forms of phyto-therapeutic intervention for the prevention and treatment of PD. Among these phytochemicals is the trans-isomer of the polyphenol, resveratrol (RES), which has been reported to alleviate many inflammatory conditions, including those associated with PD. RES has also demonstrated favorable synergistic effects on inflammation when combined with other bioactive plant-based compounds such as curcumin [28].

2. Attenuation of the Dysbiotic biofilm by RES

Since PD is initiated by a dysbiotic biofilm, modulation of the oral microbial ecosystem is a viable upstream therapeutic approach. Also, the reduction of pathogenic microbial load is a logical and necessary start to treatment, which is the primary intent of SRP and CC (www.NHS.uk; www.ADA.org).

Studies assessing the potential for addressing the pathogenic oral biofilm, reported that RES demonstrated antimicrobial action against PD pathogens. For example, O'Connor and colleagues conducted an in vitro study on different prokaryotic and eukaryotic microbes using the gold standard antiseptic rinse used in dentistry, chlorohexidine (CHX), as a positive control. They tested the inhibitory effect of RES on 15 different microbial species and only *A. actinomycetemcomitans* (*Aa*) and *P. gingivalis* (*Pg*) (ATCC2533277) showed sensitivity to RES. The authors also pointed out that the other 13 microbes were aerobic, suggesting that RES is specifically antimicrobial to anaerobes. In fact, *Pg* showed a much higher sensitivity to RES than Aa did in this study, suggesting that *Pg* may be especially vulnerable to RES, for reasons other than its anaerobic nature. However, since this was a study based on spectrophotometric optical density readings of broth cultures, the bacteria tested were planktonic and therefore not comparable to those participating in the biofilm seen in PD. Hence, although this study was a helpful preliminary survey, the definitive demonstration of the action of RES against *Pg in vivo*, was not solidified [29].

Interestingly, in 2019, Kugaji and colleagues assessed the effect of RES on an experimental biofilm both directly and indirectly. Firstly, direct assays were conducted via the determination of the minimal inhibitory and minimum bactericidal RES concentrations (MIC and MBC, respectively) applied to cultures of commercially available (e.g., ATCC 33277) and clinical strains (CS02) of *Pg*. Then, the calculated indices for MIC (156.25 μl/ml) and MBC (312.5 μl/ml) of RES, were applied to commercial strains of *Pg* to determine kill-time, adhesion to substrate, and morphological changes (determined by SEM). Next, RES was evaluated indirectly through the examination of the genetic expression of gingipains (i.e., Kgp and rgpA) and fimbriae (i.e., fimA), virulence factors from *Pg* that have been found to be instrumental in promoting the formation of the pathogenic biofilm in PD. The findings led the authors to conclude that RES displays antimicrobial action against keystone periodontal pathogen, *Pg*, as well as the ability to reduce the pathogenic biofilm indirectly, by decreasing the expression of its proteolytic virulence factors. It is also worth noting that in this study, the clinical *Pg* strain was more sensitive to RES than the commercially available strain. Regarding adhesion assays, the response to RES was also strain-dependent, which adds another layer of complexity regarding the *in vivo* translation of these findings [30].

Similarly, both antibacterial and anti-adherent action of RES on *Pg* (i.e., ATCC 33277) were reported by Lagha and colleagues in 2019. They determined an MIC and

MBC of 250 µL/mL and 500 µL/mL, respectively, and applied a luminescence assay as an indicator of ATP production, to show the bioactivity of the bacteria in the experimental biofilm. The calculated MIC of RES in this study reduced biofilm viability by over 50% [31].

Conversely, Millhouse and colleagues reported that RES did not demonstrate any antimicrobial action, after they developed an experimental model of a periodontal biofilm, which consisted of a co-culture of epithelial and microbes. This intricate co-culture included simulated saliva, and was designed to mimic the host-biofilm interface to assess the antimicrobial and anti-inflammatory properties of Chlorohexidine (CHX), compared with those of RES [32].

Since it has been reported that *Pg* demonstrates significant differences in genetic expression when planktonic compared to being engaged in a multispecies biofilm [33], evolving such a model is an important step toward *in vivo* translation [32].

However, the results from Milhouse et al. cannot be attributed to the co-cultured biofilm model alone because the RES was suspended in water, while the other three studies, which reported antimicrobial action from RES, used ethanol or dimethyl sulfoxide (DMSO). Hence, the comparability between the studies is diminished by the fact that RES has virtually no solubility in water, while DMSO and ethanol are more successful as solvents [34], but often have unpredictable biological effects of their own, which must be appropriately controlled for.

Further to this, an *in vivo* study conducted by Cirano and colleagues, employed a modified ligature-induced rat model to evaluate the action of RES against key pathogens, *Pg*, T. forsythia (*Tf*) and *Aa*. This study applied ligatures pre-treated with the individual pathogens and evaluated the antimicrobial action of RES using RT PCR of all three microbial species, accompanied by a single daily gavage of a 10 mg/Kg dose of RES over a 30-day period. In this case, no statistically significant antimicrobial activity was demonstrated by RES. However, although the RES stock was prepared using ethanol, further dilutions were performed in water, which decreases the solubility of RES. The oral delivery route (gavage) in this study suggests that low oral bioavailability [35] and instability [34] of RES may have affected the results. Consequently, the authors recognize that for future studies, applying RES via topical/transmucosal administration in the *in vivo* models may overcome this limitation [36].

Although these studies cannot definitively conclude that RES demonstrates antimicrobial activity *in vivo*, further studies may bring to light the antimicrobial status of RES, as more information emerges about the oral microbiome and the mechanisms of the intercellular interactions that govern dysbiotic biofilm formation. What is clear from this analysis is that more consideration needs to be given to the solubility, formulation, and route of delivery of RES. Indeed, *in vivo* experimental designs may benefit from routes of administration of RES that bypass its low bioavailability and stability, as new models are evolved that provide more consistent and translatable data.

3. Modulation of host immune response by RES

Investigations using ligature-induced PD animal models, have consistently reported the favorable modification of many pro-inflammatory markers as well as the reduction and/or arrest of tissue destruction. **Table 1** outlines the results of a collection of animal studies and the molecules affected by RES [28, 37–46].

Inflammatory Mediator and RES Action on Mediator	Action of Molecule	Formulation and Administration of RES	Type of Assay Used to Detect the Inflammatory Mediator/Marker	Tissue Sampled
IL-1β Decreased	Pro-inflammatory	Gavage 10 mg/Kg in 2% EtOH [37] PO 10 mg/Kg *Melinjo* seed extract [38] Gavage 20 mg/Kg [39]	RT-PCR [37] RT-PCR [38] RT-PCR [39]	Gingival tissue [37] Gingival tissue [38] Gingival tissue [39]
IL-4 Increased	Anti-inflammatory	Gavage 10 mg/Kg in Tween-80 /ddH2O [28] Gavage 10 mg/Kg in Tween-80/ddH2O [40] Gavage 10 mg/Kg in Tween 80/ddH2O [41]	ELISA [28] ELISA [40] ELISA [41]	Gingival tissue [28] Gingival tissue / Blood [40] Gingival tissue [41]
IL-6 Decreased	Pro-inflammatory	Into socket 50 μM in 0.1% DMSO [42] Gavage 10 mg/kg in 2% EtOH [37] PO 10 mg/Kg *Melinjo* seed extract [38] Gavage 20 mg/Kg [39]	Immunohistochemistry [42] RT-PCR [37] RT-PCR [38] RT-PCR [39]	Periodontium [42] Gingival tissue [37] Gingival tissue [38] Gingival tissue [39]
IL-8 Decreased	Pro-inflammatory	Gavage 20 mg/Kg [39] diabetic mice	RT-PCR [39]	Gingival tissue [39]
IL-17 Decreased	Pro-inflammatory	Gavage 10 mg/Kg in EtOH/ddH2O [43]	ELISA [43]	Gingival tissue [43]
TNF-α Decreased	Pro-inflammatory	Into socket 50 μM in 0.1% DMSO [42] Gavage 10 mg/kg in 2% EtOH [37] PO 10 mg/Kg *Melinjo* seed extract [38] Gavage 20 mg/Kg [39]	Immunohistochemistry [42] RT-PCR [37] RT-PCR [38] Serological [39]	Gingival tissue [37, 42] Gingival tissue [38] Blood [39]
IFN-γ Decreased	Pro-inflammatory	Gavage 10 mg/Kg in Tween-80 /ddH2O [28]	ELISA [28]	Gingival tissue [28]
RF Decreased	Pro-inflammatory	Gavage 10 mg/Kg in Tween-80/ddH2O [40]	ELISA [40]	Blood [40]
SOD Increased	Antioxidant	Gingival injection/5 mg/kg in DMSO [44] Gavage 10 mg/kg in Tween –80 [45]	Serological [44] ELISA [45]	Blood [44] Gingival tissue [45]
HO-1 Increased	ROS/RNS stress defense	Gingival injection/5 mg/kg in DMSO [44]	Western Blot [44] Immunohistochemistry [44]	Periodontium [44]
COX-2 Decreased	Pro-inflammatory	Gingival injection/5 mg/kg in DMSO [44]	Immunohistochemistry [44]	Periodontium [44]

Inflammatory Mediator and RES Action on Mediator	**Action of Molecule**	**Formulation and Administration of RES**	**Type of Assay Used to Detect the Inflammatory Mediator/Marker**	**Tissue Sampled**
MMP-2 Decreased	Destructive protease	Gingival injection/5 mg/kg in DMSO [44]	Immunohistochemistry [44]	Periodontium [44]
MMP-9 Decreased	Destructive protease	Gingival injection/5 mg/kg in DMSO [44]	Immunohistochemistry [44]	Periodontium [44]
Nrf2 Increased	Antioxidant	Gingival injection/5 mg/kg in DMSO [44] PO 10 mg/Kg *Melinjo* seed extract [38]	Western Blot [44] Immunohistochemistry [44] RT-PCR [38]	Periodontium [44] Gingival tissue [38]
SIRT-1 Increased	Antioxidant	Gavage 10 mg/Kg in Tween-80/ddH2O [45] PO 10 mg/Kg *Melinjo* seed extract in [38]	RT-PCR [45] RT-PCR and Western blot [38]	Gingival tissue [45] Gingival tissue [38]
ACCPA Decreased	Destructive protease Antibody	Gavage 10 mg/Kg in Tween-80/ddH2O [40]	ELISA [40]	Blood and Gingival tissue [40]
NADPH-OX Decreased	Source of ROS damage	Gavage 10 mg/Kg in Tween-80/ddH2O [45] Gavage 10 mg/Kg in Tween-80/ddH2O [46]	ELISA [45] ELISA [46]	Gingival tissue [45] Gingival tissue [46]
NF-κB Decreased	Pro-inflammatory Transcription Factor	PO 10 mg/Kg *Melinjo* seed extract [38] Gavage 20 mg/Kg [39]	RT-PCR [38] Western blot [39]	Gingival tissue [38, 39]
NQO-1 Increased	Anti-oxidant gene	PO 10 mg/Kg *Melinjo* seed extract [38]	RT-PCR [38]	Gingival tissue [38]
AMPK Induced Phosphorylation	Anti-inflammatory	PO 10 mg/Kg *Melinjo* seed extract [38]	Western blot [38]	Gingival tissue [38]
P38/MAPK Decreased Phosphorylation	Pro-inflammatory	PO 10 mg/Kg *Melinjo* seed extract [38] Gavage 20 mg/Kg [39]	Western blot [38] Western blot [39]	Gingival tissue [38] Gingival tissue [39]
STAT3 Decreased Phosphorylation	Possible Inducer of Diabetic PD	Gavage 20 mg/Kg [39]	Western blot [39]	Gingival tissue [39]
p65/NF-κB Decreased Phosphorylation	Pro-inflammatory Transcription Factor	Gavage 20 mg/Kg [39]	Western blot [39]	Gingival tissue [39]
Inos Decreased	Pro-inflammatory	PO 10 mg/Kg *Melinjo* seed extract [38]	RT-PCR [38]	Gingival tissue [38]
8-OHdG Decreased	Oxidative stress marker	PO 10 mg/Kg *Melinjo* seed extract [38]	ELISA [38]	Urine [38]
Dityrosine Decreased	Oxidative stress marker	PO 10 mg/Kg *Melinjo* seed extract in [38]	ELISA [38]	Urine [38]

Inflammatory Mediator and RES Action on Mediator	Action of Molecule	Formulation and Administration of RES	Type of Assay Used to Detect the Inflammatory Mediator/Marker	Tissue Sampled
RANKL Decreased	Increases bone resorption	Gavage 10 mg/kg in 2% EtOH [37] Gavage 10 mg/Kg in Tween-80/ddH2O [41]	RT-PCR [37] RT-PCR [41]	Gingival tissue [37] Gingival tissue [41]
NOx Decreased	Nitrosative stress marker	PO 10 mg/Kg *Melinjo* seed extract [38]	Serological [38]	Serum [38]
Nitrotyrosine Decreased	Nitrosative stress marker	PO 10 mg/Kg *Melinjo* seed extract in [38]	ELISA [38]	Serum [38]
RUNX-2 Decreased	Osteoblastic marker	Into socket 50 μM in 0.1% DMSO [42]	Immuno-histochemistry [42]	Periodontium [42]
OCN Increased	Osteoblastic hormone	Into socket 50 μM in 0.1% DMSO [42]	Immuno-histochemistry [42]	Periodontium [42]
Ki67 Decreased	Proliferation	Into socket 50 μM in 0.1% DMSO [42]	Immuno-histochemistry {37}	Periodontium [42]

Table 1.
Ligature-induced PD studies with the RES formulation, type of assay and tissue sampled for the inflammation-mediating molecules examined.

Moreover, several reports from *in vitro* studies have also reliably concluded that RES mitigates the dysregulated immune response seen in PD [47, 48]. For example, a study by Qu et al. used *Porphyromonas endodontalis* (Pe)LPS-challenged osteoblast-like mouse cells (MC3T3-E1) to identify the role of silent mating type information regulation 2 homolog 1 (SIRT-1) in the resolution of inflammation and mitigation of bone loss. Their model employed the transfection of the cells with SIRT-1 siRNA, as well as the use of SIRT-1 inhibitor, EX-527, to silence SIRT-1 activity, whilst RES was used as a SIRT-1 activator [49].

Notably, elevated levels of matrix metaloprteinase-13 (MMP-13) expression, as determined by RT-PCR, ELISA and Western blot, were evidenced upon induction by LPS. Furthermore, this induction was increased by knockdown of SIRT-1 activity, either by use of siRNA SIRT-1, or by the addition of the inhibitor, EX-527. However, pre-treatment with RES (50 μM, no solvent was specified) for 1 hour, significantly ($p < 0.05$) suppressed the mRNA expression (as determined by RT-PCR) and protein production (assayed by Western blotting and ELISA) of MMP-13 in the LPS-challenged cells. A chromatin immunoprecipitation assay (ChIP) then determined that SIRT-1 prevents the activation-stimulating binding of NFkB-p65 to the MMP-13 promoter [49], which aligns with the findings reporting RES as a SIRT-1 activator [50–52].

An early human *in vitro* study reported the use of RT-PCR and ELISA, to determine that RES decreased the mRNA levels of a range of cytokines regarded to be proinflammatory, including IL-1β, IL-6, IL-8, IL-12 and TNF-α, in *Pg* lipopolysaccharide-(LPS)-challenged human periodontal ligamental cells. The effect was reported to be both dose-(25 μM, 50 μM and 100 μM) and time-(0–72 hrs) dependent [53].

Similarly, more recent *in vitro* studies employing ELISA, found that RES significantly decreased IL-6 and IL-8, in human gingival fibroblasts (HGFs) that were stimulated by LPS [26, 54]. RES was also combined with the triterpene, Celastrol

(CEL), and loaded into a collagen film to enhance the effectiveness of coated dental implants by Wang et al. [55]. Using SEM and histochemistry, it was determined that the RES-loaded collagen films stimulated the most proliferation of the human periodontal ligamental fibroblasts (HPLFs), whilst the CEL-loaded films, demonstrated the lowest bone marrow macrophage-mediated osteogenesis. Hence, it was suggested that using both RES and CEL in the collagen film was a promising approach to the development of an efficacious dental regenerative agent [55].

In 2020, Ashour et al., used Hesperetin (HESP) as a glyoxalase 1(Glo1) inducer to assess its modulation of the damage caused to HPLFs from high glucose. This experimental *in vitro* model showed that HPLFs overloaded with glucose, increased the cellular concentration of methylglyoxal (MG) and its modified proteins, which resulted in HPLF dysfunction and inability to bind to collagen-I. By adding RES (10 μM) to the HESP, the dysfunction was corrected through the attenuation of deregulated glucose metabolism [56].

An additional study compared the anti-inflammatory activity of Tetracycline (TC), Minocycline (MC), Quercetin (QU), and RES, in LPS-stimulated macrophage-like mouse cells, (RAW264.7). Upon the application of differential scanning calorimetry, and RT-PCR, the anti-inflammatory activity was determined as an index of COX-2 inhibition and it was concluded that the order from highest anti-inflammatory action to lowest was as follows: QU > RES > MC > TC [57].

4. Restoration of damaged periodontal tissues by RES

An extensive *in vitro* and *in situ* investigation by Wang et al., using human periodontal ligamental stem cells (HPLSCs) treated with TNF-α, found that RES conserved their osteo-differentiation. Here, histological analysis showed that RES preserved the formation of cell aggregates and made the cells more resilient to TNF-α—induced inhibition of alkaline phosphatase (PhoA) whilst promoting mineralization. Further to this, RT-PCR was used to show the partial restoration of mRNA expression of the osteo-differentiation drivers, OCN, RUNX2, PhoA and Collagen-1. Moreover, Western blotting showed restored values for OCN, Collagen-1, and RUNX2, an osteoblastic modulator, confirming the mRNA findings at the level of protein. The *in vitro* action of RES on the ontogenetic capabilities of HPLSCs originating from PD patients was also determined to be beneficial through histological analysis, RT-PCR and Western blot. Additionally, an ectopic regeneration experiment was conducted, involving transplantation of normal, PD alone, or RES-treated PD-induced HPLSC aggregates into nude mice, which allowed the researchers to assess the regenerative action of RES *in situ* [58].

An additional *in vitro* study on HPLSCs, employing histochemical analysis, RT-PCR, Western blot, as well as ELISA, reported that the osteogenic suppression induced by treatment with TNF-α was mitigated by RES. Also, the results of ERK1/2 pathway inhibition and activation assays showed that the anti-inflammatory action of RES was diminished by ERK1/2 pathway inhibition. This suggests that the mechanism employed by RES, involves activation of the ERK1/2 pathway in TNF-α-challenged HPLSCs [59].

Interestingly, Kudo et al., examined the role of SIRT1 in angiogenesis in PD by treating human umbilical vein endothelial cells (HUVECs) with *E. coli* LPS plus RES (i.e., a SIRT1 activator) or sirtinol (i.e., a SIRT1 inhibitor). Also, in this study, periapical granulomas were obtained from PD patients, whereas healthy individuals provided normal periodontal tissues, which were also assayed. Immunofluorescent imaging using antibodies against SIRT1 and Ki67, showed that the periapical granulomas had higher expression of both SIRT1 and Ki67, compared to healthy gingival tissue. Additionally, the quantification of the mRNA of SIRT1, VEGF (which stimulates endothelial growth and differentiation into vessel morphology) and VE-cadherin (an adhesion protein for endothelia) in the LPS-induced HUVECS indicated that the mRNA expression statistically increased for all three proteins ($P = 0.0019$ (SIRT-1), 0.00005(VEGF) and 0.0045 (VE-cadherin)) in the RES-treated groups compared to the group treated with sirtinol [60].

5. Mitigation of systemic conditions associated with PD by RES

Studies have been conducted integrating RA, DM, cigarette smoking or osteoporosis (OP) into their induced-PD models. For example, two studies employed a ligature-induced PD rat model which incorporated three, eight-minute exposures per day, to the equivalent of 10 cigarettes, for 37 days, and examined the effects of RES on bone loss and oxidative stress, respectively [40, 41]. In this study, they found that the gingival tissue of the RES-treated group displayed higher expression of anti-inflammatory cytokine IL-4, and the antioxidant SIRT-1 [40], suggesting that RES plays a beneficial role when the added risk factor of smoking is involved. Further to this, RT-PCR determined that the mRNA expression of the osteoclastic inducer, RANKL was diminished by RES [41] and ELISA showed that the ROS inducer, NADPH oxidase, was also significantly diminished in the RES-treated group (i.e., RES + Cigarette Smoke) whilst SOD was significantly higher ($p < 0.05$) (**Table 1**) [37].

Moreover, the administration of RES was found to decrease the TH17/TH2 cell ratio in diseased gingival tissue, suggesting that it may modulate the overstimulation of TH17 (i.e., TH lymphocytes purported be stimulated by the outer membrane protein of *Pg*) production, which contributes to tissue destruction [38, 61]. These results also indicate that RES may assist in the mitigation of the periodontal damage contributed to, by the modifiable risk factor, smoking [38]. Additionally, a study which assessed the effect of RES on experimental PD in diabetic mice, found that RES decreased the mRNA expression of LPS—induced inflammatory cytokines IL-1β, IL-6, IL-8 and TNF-α. In addition, the LPS-induced phosphorylation, and therefore activation, of transcription factors downstream to TLR4, p65 NF-κB, p38 MAPK, and STAT3, was also suppressed by RES, suggesting that RES works through the TLR4 signaling pathway [39]. Moreover, RES was also found to reduce alveolar bone loss and attenuate hyperglycemia [39, 56], demonstrating its potential as an attenuator of diabetic PD.

An additional study conducted by Correa and colleagues, examined the effect of RES compared to Ibuprofen on experimental PD and RA combined, using the ligature-induced PD rat model. Here, they determined by way of ELISA, that the administration RES or Ibuprofen resulted in the reduction of anti-cyclic citrullinated peptide antibody (ACCPA) in the tissues by 72% and 99%, respectively ($p < 0.05$), and, RES alone was reported to reduce serum rheumatoid factor (RF)($p < 0.05$). In this study, RES also demonstrated sustained reduction in paw edema compared to Ibuprofen. Moreover, the RES treated group demonstrated reduced articular damage in the histological analysis, indicating its ability to modulate RA-induced damage in the context of experimental PD in rats [40].

Similarly, in an animal study, using ovariectomized rats and PD-induction via ligature installment, RES was compared to Zoledronate, a drug used to treat osteoporosis (OP). Here, ELISA showed that RES downregulated NADPH oxidase and reduced alveolar bone loss, but not as drastically as in the Zoledronate-treated group. Nonetheless, the results suggest that RES may attenuate alveolar bone loss in estrogen-deficient rats via the attenuation of NADPH oxidase, making NADPH oxidase a potential drug target for RES. Using a human *in vitro* neuroinflammation model, it was determined that several pathways that promote oxidative stress (via the decrease in AKT1, FOS, IKBKB, IRF1, JAK2, NFKB1PIK3RI, RELA, STAT1, TNF-α and TNFRSF1 mRNA) as well as iNOS (via the decrease in FOS, IKBKB, IRAK1, IRAK2, IRF1, JAK2, NFKB1, RELA and STAT1 mRNA) was attenuated by RES. The researchers in this study used qPCR and biochemical pathway analysis to examine 96 genes, present in human neuroblastoma cells, that were induced into inflammation via the application of LPS originating from *Pg*. It was concluded that RES decreased NF-κB-mediated acute inflammation pathways in human neuroblastoma cell culture. Further to this, RES was also reported to inhibit IGF-1 and Insulin receptor while activating the PTEN, PPARa/RXRa, PPAR metabolic pathways. This extensive *in vitro* study showed the potential for RES to address Pg-related disease, with a particular focus on the prevention of AD [62].

6. Clinical translation of RES

Two randomized clinical trials were conducted by Javid et al. (IRCT ID: IRCT2015012420765N1). One study evaluated the effect of RES on blood glucose, Insulin, Insulin resistance and periodontal markers in 43 type two DM patients aged 30–60 years old, with chronic moderate PD. This double-blind and placebo-controlled study, evaluated the impact of RES by supplementing the experimental group with 480 mg capsules containing RES, once a day, for 28 days. The subjects in the placebo group were given identical capsules containing 480 mg of starch. Although no significant differences in fasting blood glucose or TGs between the groups were evident, the RES-supplemented group showed significantly lower ($p < 0.05$) periodontal pocket depth, serum fasting glucose and insulin resistance [63].

The second study, also a randomized clinical trial, assessed the serum levels of inflammatory cytokines IL-6 and TNF-α, as well as total antioxidant capacity (TAC) and clinical attachment loss (CAL) in 43 patients with type two DM and PD. After 28 days of supplementation with 480 mg/d of RES, serum levels of IL-6 were significantly lower($p = 0.039$), but the other parameters measured, showed no significant change compared to control [64]. The results of both studies do not fully align with those of the animal studies, which may be partly due to the formulation and posology used. That is, Javid et al., applied a 480 mg capsule of *Polygonum cuspidatum* reported to contain 240 mg of RES. In general, the animal studies used 10–20 mg/kg of pure RES, delivered via gavage, which would calibrate to approximately 730–1460 mg of RES in this study, considering the average mass of the human subjects in the RES-treated group (mean mass of subjects =73.8 ± 10.2 Kg) [63, 64].

Lastly, Shoukheba, conducted a six-month human study in 2020 consisting of 15 male smokers with moderate to severe (i.e., CAL >5 mm) PD, following SRP. Interestingly, RES gel (0.001% w/v final concentration) was directly applied to the testing sites (15 healthy, 15 with PD), applying the split mouth method at days 7,14, and 21. The clinical parameters, plaque index (PI), probing pocket depth (PPD), bleeding index (BI)and CAL were assessed. In addition, the gingival crevicular fluid was collected during the treatment visits to assess SOD levels. The SOD levels were higher in the RES group compared to control and although both groups showed a significant decrease ($p < 0.05$) in the clinical parameters, PPD and CAL, at the three-month mark, only the RES-treated group demonstrated significant improvement from baseline at 6 months ($p < 0.05$) [65].

Again, further studies using RES in the absence of SRP, need to be conducted to fully elucidate the role of RES in the attenuation of PD. In addition to this, since cigarette smokers have been reported to have higher susceptibility to an oral Pg infection (Zeller et al., 2014), perhaps more information may be gained by comparing the Pg load between groups [65].

RES has a long-term body of evidence reporting its low bioavailability, which is mainly due to its physicochemical properties. That is, RES is pH-, thermo-, and photo-sensitive, [66]. More importantly, RES is unstable under physiological pH (7.4) and temperature (37°C), thus diminishing the *in vivo* translatability [67–69].

There are a myriad of studies demonstrating the effective mitigation of the low bioavailability, stability and pharmacokinetic profile of RES via nano-formulation. In this way, RES may be potentially upgraded from a supplement to a nanomedicine.

7. Improvement of RES as a therapeutic via nanotechnology

Nanotechnology, which employs materials that measure at <100 nm in at least one dimension, has been found to improve the stability, bioavailability and activity of RES. Overall, there exist several studies exploring the action of various formulations of Nano-RES which reported improvements in stability, bioavailability and pharmacokinetics, compared to RES in bulk form [70–75]. For example, nano-formulations employing solid lipid nanoparticles (SLNs) and nanostructured lipid carriers (NLCs), are purported to have higher stability, and a pharmacokinetic profile indicative of sustained release. Interestingly, SLNs and NLCs have more economical scalability compared to liposomal systems [70], making them attractive options as RES carriers.

Successful production of the SLNs and NLCs may be accomplished using waxes, fats, oils, or combinations thereof, combined with surfactant, and the application of high-pressure shear homogenization [71], sonication [72] and [73], or both [74, 75]. Studies involving RES-loaded SLNs and NLCs, demonstrated higher stability compared to bulk RES, as indicated by the high zeta potentials reported (i.e., $\zeta > 20$ mV, [74] and $\zeta < -20$ mV, [71–73, 75]).

Furthermore, Singh and Pai reported a self-nano-emulsifying drug delivery system (SNEDDS) that enhanced the pharmacokinetic profile of RES *in vivo*. Here, the RES-loaded SNEDDS was administered orally to rats (at 20 mg/Kg body weight dose) before withdrawing serial aliquots of blood. The SNEDDS was designed to automatically form a nano-emulsion once in contact with the fluids of the gastrointestinal tract and spontaneous emulsification into stable ($\zeta = -29.76$ mV), 57 nm nano-globules took place in 43 seconds after being placed in 0.1 M HCl. The authors noted that the enhanced oral availability of RES-loaded SNEDDS compared to crude RES was likely due to an increase in absorbability as well as diminished first pass clearing by the liver enzyme CYP3A4 [76].

Moreover, Al-Bishri and colleagues compared the anti-diabetic activity of a commercial nano-emulsion of RES (Life Enhancement, Petaluma, California, USA) with that of chromium picolinate in streptozocin-induced diabetic in rats. Two weeks after the induction of DM, rats in the experimental groups were orally administered either (80 μg/Kg body weight) or Nano-RES emulsion (20 μg/Kg body weight) every day for 30 days when serum levels for glucose insulin, as well as biomarkers: NO, SOD, CAT, GPX, GST and GSH were determined. Both nano-RES emulsion and Chromium picolinate demonstrated inhibition of the oxidative stress induced from hyperglycemia [77].

Further to this, explorations emphasizing the fortification process involved in functional food production, demonstrate the potential of functional foods to be administered as an effective prevention, management, and treatment of PD. For example, Ahmad and Gani, assessed the biological action of RES-fortified snacks and reported that starch nano-encapsulation improved the thermostability of RES whilst enhancing anti-diabetic and anti-obesity effects compared to bulk RES, which was determined by the percent inhibition of the enzymes: α-glucosidase and, pancreatic lipase, and cholesterol esterase, respectively [78]. Inhibition of lipid peroxidase, which was also reported, demonstrated antioxidant activity of the nano-formulated food complex. Moreover, since the nano-embedded RES-fortified designer food-snacks exhibited enhanced desired activity at physiological pH (7.4) and temperature (37°C) the formulation in this study shows promise as a functional food [78].

Similarly, Jayan et al. reported the sustained release of RES from ZEIN-encapsulated nanoparticles (NPs) under physiological conditions (i.e., pH 7.4, 37°C) [79] and casein-encapsulated RES NPs, designed by Penlava et al., were found to be stable through a continuous pH range mimicking those of the gastrointestinal compartments (i.e., pH 1.2 for 2 hours and pH 6.8 for 2–24 hours). Interestingly, the latter study also demonstrated in vivo (using rats), a ten-fold increase in oral availability of casein-nano-encapsulated RES compared to the bulk form as determined by blood plasma assays over a 24-hour period following a single oral dose of 15 mg/Kg of RES (in ddH2O and PEG) or Casein-encapsulated RES NPs [80].

Additionally, Rabbani and colleagues set out to explore the fortification of foods and reported that when enhanced with a nano-encapsulated formulation of RES, mayonnaise demonstrated extended shelf-life, as suggested by the reduction in peroxide value over a six-month period. The ability of the nano-RES food complex to neutralize DPPH free radicals was investigated and the initially high number of free radicals present in the mayonnaise nano-RES complex were attributed to the successful encapsulation (and therefore protection) of RES in the nano formulation. Additionally, characterization of the mayonnaise nano-RES complex was conducted using XRD and Fourier transform infrared (FTIR) spectroscopy and RES was found to be amorphous (via XRD), demonstrating its incorporation into the complex, and it was confirmed that the molecular structure of the drug was retained while interacting with the complex via hydrogen bonds (via FTIR spectroscopy) [81].

Additionally, a promising 2021 investigation by Berta et al., involved the design of an oral Nano-RES spray via encapsulation of crude RES in 2-hydroxypropyl-β-cyclodextrins (i.e., RES-HPβCD) and tested its action on plaque formation in children. This study demonstrated that after using the spray once per day, the RES-HPβCD plaque was significantly reduced; the spray was also found to be doubled in efficacy when compared to tooth brushing alone [82].

8. From trash to treasure: Sources of trans-RES

RES is widely known in the Western hemisphere as a product from the skin of red grapes but there are other viable sources. In fact, the most abundant source of RES is found in roots of the plant, *P. cuspidatum* (i.e., Japanese knotweed), which has been used for a while in the East as a Traditional Chinese Medicine (i.e., ko-jo-kon) for the treatment of ailments such as cardiovascular disease. Unfortunately, this valuable resource has been wasted in the West, where it is perceived as an invasive species to be burned and buried. Since Japanese knotweed is edible and consists of more than 90% RES, adjustments to the current perception of the plant, could benefit many, as awareness of its medicinal (and potentially economic) value has been surfacing in the western scientific literature over recent decades [83].

Commercially available micronized versions of pure RES powder have been available for purchase for some time (e.g., www.megaresveratrol.net and www.Biotivia.com). However, nano-formulations of RES for oral use (many are topical [84]) have just began to emerge within the last year (e.g., www.oic.com.vn/en/ (Vietnam) www.nanoceuticalsolutions.com (USA), and www.hiimmune.com/product/nano-resveratrol-30ml/ (UK)).

9. Conclusion

According to the body of evidence explored in this chapter, the future of Nano-RES as a viable medicine for the prevention, management and treatment of PD and its associated systemic diseases, is promising.

In addition to nanomedicines for treatment, the development of functional foods fortified with Nano-RES, which demonstrate the potential for the preventative measures, may be an important addition to our dietary regimen moving forward [85].

Further to this, to realize the full potential of Nano-RES, an initiative is needed, to encourage more clinical research on the efficacy of low-cost, phytonutrient-based, novel nano-formulations, specifically aimed to address PD.

This could result in the commercial availability of high quality, ubiquitously accessible, effective RES-based Nano-formulations, and ultimately, a step toward a healthier future population.

Author details

Tracey Lynn Harney[1,2,3]

1 Nanotechnology for Medicine and Health Care, University of Oxford, UK

2 United States of Consciousness Ltd, Bermuda

3 Department of Biology, Bermuda College, Paget, Bermuda

*Address all correspondence to: tharney@college.bm

References

[1] Genco R, Sanz M. Clinical and public health implications of periodontal and systemic diseases: An overview. Periodontology 2000. 2020;**83**(1):7-13. DOI: 10.1111/prd.12344

[2] Bernabe E, Marcenes W, Hernandez C, Bailey J, et al. Global, regional, and national levels and trends in burden of oral conditions from 1990 to 2017: A systematic analysis for the global burden of disease 2017 study. Journal of Dental Research. 2020;**99**(4):362-373. DOI: 10.1177/0022034520908533

[3] Frencken J, Sharma P, Stenhouse L, Green D, et al. Global epidemiology of dental caries and severe periodontitis—A comprehensive review. Journal of Clinical Periodontology. 2017;**44**:94-105. DOI: 10.3390/ma13112631

[4] Tonetti M, Jepsen S, Jin L, Otomo-Corgel J. Impact of the global burden of periodontal diseases on health, nutrition and wellbeing of mankind: A call for global action. Journal of Clinical Periodontology. 2017;**44**(5):456-462

[5] Agarwal S. Impact of periodontitis on cardiovascular diseases. European Journal of Dental and Oral Health. 2021;**2**(2):1-8. DOI: 10.24018/EJDENT.2021.2.2.48

[6] Bengtsson V, Persson G, Berglund J, Renvert S. Periodontitis related to cardiovascular events and mortality: A long-time longitudinal study. Clinical Oral Investigations. 2021;**25**(6):4085-4095. DOI: 10.1007/s00784-020-03739-x

[7] Bodanese L, Louzeiro G, Magnus G, Baptista Â, et al. Association between periodontitis and myocardial infarction: Systematic review and meta-analysis. International Journal of Cardiovascular Sciences. 2021;**34**(5Supl.1):121-127

[8] Sia S, Jan M, Wang Y, Huang Y, Wei J. Periodontitis is associated with incidental valvular heart disease: A nationwide population-based cohort study. Journal of Clinical Periodontology. 2021;**48**(8):1085-1092

[9] Surma S, Romańczyk M, Witalińska-Łabuzek J, Czerniuk M, et al. Periodontitis, blood pressure, and the risk and control of arterial hypertension: Epidemiological, clinical, and pathophysiological aspects—Review of the literature and clinical trials. Current Hypertension Reports. 2021;**23**(5). Available from: https://link.springer.com/article/10.1007/s11906-021-01140-x [Accessed: 28 October 2022]

[10] Tiensripojamarn N, Lertpimonchai A, Tavedhikul K, Udomsak A, et al. Periodontitis is associated with cardiovascular diseases: A 13-year study. Journal of Clinical Periodontology. 2021;**48**(3):348-356

[11] Trindade F, Perpétuo L, Ferreira R, Leite-Moreira A, et al. Automatic text-mining as an unbiased approach to uncover molecular associations between periodontitis and coronary artery disease. Biomarkers. 2021;**26**(5):385-394

[12] Hajishengallis G. Interconnection of periodontal disease and comorbidities: Evidence, mechanisms, and implications. Periodontology 2000. 2022;**89**(1):9-18

[13] Chen H, Jiang W. Application of high-throughput sequencing in understanding human oral microbiome related with health and disease. Frontiers in Microbiology. 2014;**5**:1-6

[14] Kilian M, Chapple I, Hannig M, Marsh P, et al. The oral microbiome—An update for oral healthcare

professionals. British Dental Journal. 2016;**221**(10):657-666

[15] Najmanova L, Sabova L, Lenartova M, Janatova T, et al. R/G value: A numeric index of individual periodontal health and oral microbiome dynamics. Frontiers in Cellular and Infection Microbiology. 2021;**11**:1-13. DOI: 10.3389/fcimb.2021.602643

[16] Sedghi L, DiMassa V, Harrington A, Lynch S, Kapila Y. The Oral microbiome: Role of key organisms and complex networks in oral health and disease. Periodontology 2000. 2021;**87**(1):107-131

[17] Berger D, Rakhamimova A, Pollack A, Loewy Z, et al. Oral biofilms: Development, control, and analysis. High-Throughput. 2018;7(3):24. DOI: 10.3390/ht7030024

[18] Deo PN, Deshmukh R. Oral microbiome: Unveiling the fundamentals. Journal of Oral and Maxillofacial Pathology: JOMFP. 2019;**23**:122-128

[19] Radaic A, Kapila Y. The Oralome and its Dysbiosis: New insights into oral microbiome-host interactions. Computational and Structural Biotechnology Journal. 2021;**19**:1335-1360

[20] Hajishengallis G, Darveau RP, Curtis MA. The keystone-pathogen hypothesis. Nature Reviews Microbiology. 2012;**10**(10):717-725. DOI: 10.1038/nrmicro2873 [Accessed: 28 October 2022]

[21] Lunar Silva I, Cascales E. Molecular strategies underlying Porphyromonas gingivalis virulence. Journal of Molecular Biology. 2021;**433**(7):166836

[22] De Andrade K, Almeida-da-Silva C, Coutinho-Silva R. Immunological pathways triggered by porphyromonas gingivalis and fusobacterium nucleatum: Therapeutic possibilities? Mediators of Inflammation. 2019;**2019**:1-20. DOI: 10.1155/2019/7241312

[23] Matsuura M. Structural modifications of bacterial lipopolysaccharide that facilitate gram-negative bacteria evasion of host innate immunity. Frontiers in Immunology. 2013;**4**:1-9. DOI: 10.3389/fimmu.2013.00109

[24] Golub L, Lee H. Periodontal therapeutics: Current host-modulation agents and future directions. Periodontology 2000. 2019;**82**(1):186-204. DOI: 10.1111/prd.12315

[25] Gonçalves V, Musskopf M, Rivera-Concepcion A, Yu C, Wong S, Tuin S, et al. Systemic dietary hesperidin modulation of Osteoclastogenesis, bone homeostasis and periodontal disease in mice. International Journal of Molecular Sciences. 2022;**23**(13):7100

[26] Farzanegan A, Shokuhian M, Jafari S, Shirazi F, Shahidi M. Anti-histaminic effects of resveratrol and Silymarin on human gingival fibroblasts. Inflammation. 2019;**42**(5):1622-1629

[27] Asteriou E, Gkoutzourelas A, Mavropoulos A, Katsiari C, Sakkas L, BogdanosD.Curcuminforthemanagement of periodontitis and early ACPA-positive rheumatoid arthritis: Killing two birds with one stone. Nutrients. 2018;**10**(7):908

[28] Corrêa M, Pires P, Ribeiro F, Pimentel S, et al. Systemic treatment with resveratrol and/or curcumin reduces the progression of experimental periodontitis in rats. Journal of Periodontal Research. 2016;**52**(2):201-209

[29] O'Connor D, Wong R, Rabie A. Resveratrol inhibits periodontal

pathogens in vitro. Phytotherapy Research. 2011;**25**(11):1727-1731

[30] Kugaji M, Kumbar V, Peram M, Patil S, et al. Effect of resveratrol on biofilm formation and virulence factor gene expression of Porphyromonas gingivalis in periodontal disease. APMIS. 2019;**127**(4):187-195

[31] Lagha A, Andrian E, Grenier D. Resveratrol attenuates the pathogenic and inflammatory properties of Porphyromonas gingivalis. Molecular Oral Microbiology. 2019;**34**(3):118-130

[32] Millhouse E, Jose A, Sherry L, Lappin D, et al. Development of an in vitro periodontal biofilm model for assessing antimicrobial and host modulatory effects of bioactive molecules. BMC Oral Health. 2014;**14**(1):1-11

[33] Sánchez M, Romero-Lastra P, Ribeiro-Vidal H, Llama-Palacios A, et al. Comparative gene expression analysis of planktonic Porphyromonas gingivalis ATCC 33277 in the presence of a growing biofilm versus planktonic cells. BMC Microbiology. 2019;**19**(1):1-11

[34] Robinson K, Mock C, Liang D. Pre-formulation studies of resveratrol. Drug Development and Industrial Pharmacy. 2014;**41**(9):1464-1469

[35] Planas J, Alfaras I, Colom H, Juan M. The bioavailability and distribution of trans-resveratrol are constrained by ABC transporters. Archives of Biochemistry and Biophysics. 2012;**527**(2):67-73

[36] Cirano F, Casarin R, Ribeiro F, Casati M, et al. Effect of resveratrol on periodontal pathogens during experimental periodontitis in rats. Brazilian Oral Research. 2016;**30**(1). Available from: https://www.scielo.br/j/bor/a/TSWnY94YqcYT9C93MtfCbWC/?lang=en [Accessed: 28 October 2022]

[37] Chen J, Wang Y, Wang M, Wang B, et al. Resveratrol inhibited inflammation and alveolar bone loss in periodontitis. International Journal of Dentistry and Oral Science. 2015:1-5. Available from: https://www.academia.edu/19794213/Resveratrol_Inhibited_Inflammation_and_Alveolar_Bone_Loss_in_Periodontitis?auto=citations&from=cover_page. [Accessed: 5 August 2022]

[38] Tamaki N, Cristina Orihuela-Campos R, Inagaki Y, Fukui M, et al. Resveratrol improves oxidative stress and prevents the progression of periodontitis via the activation of the Sirt1/AMPK and the Nrf2/antioxidant defense pathways in a rat periodontitis model. Free Radical Biology and Medicine. 2014;**75**:22-229

[39] Zhen L, Fan D, Zhang Y, Cao X, Wang L. Resveratrol ameliorates experimental periodontitis in diabetic mice through negative regulation of TLR4 signaling. Acta Pharmacologica Sinica. 2014;**36**(2):221-228

[40] Corrêa M, Pires P, Ribeiro F, Pimentel S, et al. Systemic treatment with resveratrol reduces the progression of experimental periodontitis and arthritis in rats. PLoS One. 2018;**13**(10):204414. DOI: 10.1371/journal.pone.0204414

[41] Ribeiro F, Pino D, Franck F, Benatti B, et al. Resveratrol inhibits periodontitisrelated bone loss in rats subjected to cigarette smoke inhalation. Journal of Periodontology. 2017;**88**(8):788-798

[42] Adhikari N, Prasad Aryal Y, Jung J, Ha J, et al. Resveratrol enhances bone formation by modulating inflammation in the mouse periodontitis model. Journal of Periodontal Research. 2021;**56**(4):735-745

[43] Casati M, Algayer C, Cardoso da Cruz G, Ribeiro F, et al. Resveratrol

decreases periodontal breakdown and modulates local levels of cytokines during periodontitis in rats. Journal of Periodontology. 2013;**84**(10):58-64

[44] Bhattarai G, Poudel S, Kook S, Lee J. Resveratrol prevents alveolar bone loss in an experimental rat model of periodontitis. Acta Biomaterialia. 2016;**29**:398-408

[45] Corrêa M, Absy S, Tenenbaum H, Ribeiro F, et al. Resveratrol attenuates oxidative stress during experimental periodontitis in rats exposed to cigarette smoke inhalation. Journal of Periodontal Research. 2019;**54**(3):225-232

[46] Molez A, Nascimento E, Haiter Neto F, Cirano F, et al. Effect of resveratrol on the progression of experimental periodontitis in an Ovariectomized rat model of osteoporosis: Morphometric, immune-enzymatic, and gene expression analysis. Journal of Periodontal Research. 2020;**55**(6):840-849

[47] Calabrese E. Hormesis and dental apical papilla stem cells. Chemico-Biological Interactions. 2022;**357**:109887. DOI: 10.1016/j.cbi.2022.109887

[48] Li W, Huang X, Yu W, Xu Y, Huang R, Park J, et al. Activation of functional somatic stem cells promotes endogenous tissue regeneration. Journal of Dental Research. 2022;**101**(7):802-811

[49] Qu L, Yu Y, Qiu L, Yang D, et al. Sirtuin 1 regulates matrix metalloproteinase-13 expression induced by Porphyromonas endodontalis lipopolysaccharide via targeting nuclear factor–κB in osteoblasts. Journal of Oral Microbiology. 2017;**9**(1):1317578

[50] Borra M, Smith B, Denu J. Mechanism of human SIRT1 activation by resveratrol. Journal of Biological Chemistry. 2005;**280**(17):17187-17195

[51] Chao S, Chen Y, Huang K, Kuo K, et al. Induction of sirtuin-1 signaling by resveratrol induces human chondrosarcoma cell apoptosis and exhibits antitumor activity. Scientific Reports. 2017;**7**(1):1-11

[52] Hou X, Rooklin D, Fang H, Zhang Y. Resveratrol serves as a protein-substrate interaction stabilizer in human SIRT1 activation. Scientific Reports. 2016;**6**(1):1-9

[53] Rizzo A, Bevilacqua N, Guida L, Annunziata M, et al. Effect of resveratrol and modulation of cytokine production on human periodontal ligament cells. Cytokine. 2012;**60**(1):197-204. DOI: 10.1016/j.cyto.2012.06.004

[54] Shahidi M, Vaziri F, Haerian A, Farzanegan A, et al. Proliferative and AntiInflammatory effects of resveratrol and Silymarin on human gingival fibroblasts: A view to the future. Journal of dentistry (Tehran, Iran). 2017;**14**(4):203-211

[55] Wang R, Bao B, Bao C, Wang S, et al. Resveratrol and celastrol loaded collagen dental implants regulate periodontal ligament fibroblast growth and osteoclastogenesis of bone marrow macrophages. Chemistry & Biodiversity. 2020. [Preprint] DOI: 10.1002/cbdv.202000295

[56] Ashour A, Xue M, Al-Motawa M, Thornalley P, Rabbani N. Glycolytic overload-driven dysfunction of periodontal ligament fibroblasts in high glucose concentration, corrected by glyoxalase 1 inducer. BMJ Open Diabetes Research & Care. 2020;**8**(2):72-81

[57] Murakami Y, Kawata A, Suzuki S, Fujisawa S. Radical-scavenging and pro-anti-inflammatory activity of tetracycline and related phenolic compounds with or without visible light irradiation. In Vivo. 2019;**34**(1):81-94

[58] Wang Y, Zhao P, Sui B, Liu N, et al. Resveratrol enhances the functionality and improves the regeneration of mesenchymal stem cell aggregates. Experimental & Molecular Medicine. 2018;**50**(6):1-15

[59] Yuan J, Wang X, Ma D, Gao H, et al. Resveratrol rescues TNF-α-induced inhibition of osteogenesis in human periodontal ligament stem cells via the ERK1/2 pathway. Molecular Medicine Reports. 2020;**21**:2085-2094. DOI: 10.3892/mmr.2020.11021

[60] Kudo H, Takeichi O, Hatori K, Makino K, et al. A potential role for the silent information regulator 2 homologue 1 (SIRT1) in periapical periodontitis. International Endodontic Journal. 2018;**51**(7):747-757

[61] Tesmer L, Lundy S, Sarkar S, Fox D. Th17 cells in human disease. Immunological Reviews. 2008;**223**(1):87-113

[62] Bahar B, Singhrao S. An evaluation of the molecular mode of action of transresveratrol in the Porphyromonas gingivalis lipopolysaccharide challenged neuronal cell model. Molecular Biology Reports. 2020;**48**(1):147-156

[63] Javid A, Hormoznejad R, Yousefimanesh H, Zakerkish M, et al. The impact of resveratrol supplementation on blood glucose, insulin, insulin resistance, triglyceride, and periodontal markers in type 2 diabetic patients with chronic periodontitis. Phytotherapy Research. 2016;**31**(1):108-114

[64] Javid A, Hormoznejad R, Yousefimanesh H, Haghighi-zadeh M, Zakerkish M. Impact of resveratrol supplementation on inflammatory, antioxidant, and periodontal markers in type 2 diabetic patients with chronic periodontitis. Diabetes & Metabolic Syndrome: Clinical Research & Reviews. 2019;**13**(4):769-2774

[65] Shoukheba M. Effect of resveratrol as an antioxidant in the treatment of smoker patients with stage III periodontitis. SAR Journal of Dentistry, Oral Surgery and Medicine. 2020;**1**(7):1-7. Available from: http://www.sarmedjournals.com/media/articles/SARJDOSM_11_1-7.pdf. [Accessed: 3 August 2022]

[66] Zupančič Š, Lavrič Z, Kristl J. Stability and solubility of trans-resveratrol are strongly influenced by pH and temperature. European Journal of Pharmaceutics and Biopharmaceutics. 2015;**93**:196-204

[67] Singh C, Ndiaye M, Ahmad N. Resveratrol and cancer: Challenges for clinical translation. Biochimica et Biophysica Acta (BBA)—Molecular Basis of Disease. 2015;**1852**(6):1178-1185

[68] Smoliga J, Vang O, Baur J. Challenges of translating basic research into therapeutics: Resveratrol as an example. The Journals of Gerontology Series A: Biological Sciences and Medical Sciences. 2011;**67A**(2):158-167

[69] Subramanian L, Youssef S, Bhattacharya S, Kenealey J, et al. Resveratrol: Challenges in translation to the clinic—A critical discussion. Clinical Cancer Research. 2010;**16**(24):5942-5948

[70] Naseri N, Valizadeh H, Zakeri-Milani P. Solid lipid nanoparticles and nanostructured lipid carriers: Structure, preparation and application. Advanced Pharmaceutical Bulletin. 2015;**5**(3):305-313

[71] Soeratri W, Hidayah R, Rosita N. Effect of combination soy bean oil and oleic acid to characteristic, penetration, physical stability of nanostructure

lipid carrier resveratrol. Folia Medica Indonesiana. 2019;**55**(3):213

[72] Poonia N, Kaur Narang J, Lather V, Beg S, Sharma T, Singh B, et al. Resveratrol loaded functionalized nanostructured lipid carriers for breast cancer targeting: Systematic development, characterization and pharmacokinetic evaluation. Colloids and Surfaces B: Biointerfaces. 2019;**181**:756-766

[73] Qin L, Lu T, Qin Y, He Y, Cui N, et al. In vivo effect of resveratrol-loaded solid lipid nanoparticles to relieve physical fatigue for sports nutrition supplements. Molecules. 2020;**25**(22):5302. DOI: 10.3390/molecules25225302

[74] Midha K, Nagpal N, Polonini, et al. Nano delivery systems of resveratrol to enhance its Oral bioavailability. American Journal of Pharmacy and Health Research. 2015;**3**(7). Available from: https://www.researchgate.net/publication/281062873_Nano_delivery_Systems_of_Resveratrol_to_Enhance_its_Oral_Bioavailability. [Accessed: 3 August 2022]

[75] Zu Y, Overby H, Ren G, Fan Z, et al. Resveratrol liposomes and lipid Nanocarriers: Comparison of characteristics and inducing browning of white adipocytes. Colloids and Surfaces B: Biointerfaces. 2018;**164**:414-423

[76] Singh G, Pai R. Trans-resveratrol self-nano-emulsifying drug delivery system (SNEDDS) with enhanced bioavailability potential: Optimization, pharmacokinetics and in situ single pass intestinal perfusion (spip) studies. Drug Delivery. 2014;**22**(4):522-530

[77] Al-Bishri W. Attenuating impacts of chromium and nano resveratrol against hyperglycemia induced oxidative stress in diabetic rat. International Journal of Pharmaceutical Research & Allied Sciences. 2017;**6**(2):61-69

[78] Ahmad M, Gani A. Development of novel functional snacks containing nanoencapsulated resveratrol with anti-diabetic, anti-obesity and antioxidant properties. Food Chemistry. 2021;**352**:129-323

[79] Jayan H, Maria Leena M, Sivakama Sundari S, et al. Improvement of bioavailability for resveratrol through encapsulation in zein using electrospraying technique. Journal of Functional Foods. 2019;**57**:417-424

[80] Peñalva R, Morales J, González-Navarro C, Larrañeta E, et al. Increased oral bioavailability of resveratrol by its encapsulation in casein nanoparticles. International Journal of Molecular Sciences. 2018;**19**(9):2816

[81] Rabbani M, Pezeshki A, Ahmadi R, Mohammadi M, et al. Phytosomal Nanocarriers for encapsulation and delivery of resveratrol: Preparation, characterization, and application in mayonnaise. LWT. 2021;**151**:112093. DOI: 10.1016/j.jphotobiol.2020.111846

[82] Berta G, Romano F, Vallone R, Abbadessa G, et al. An innovative strategy for oral biofilm control in early childhood based on a resveratrol-cyclodextrin nanotechnology approach. Materials. 2021;**14**(14):3801. DOI: 10.3390/ma14143801

[83] Chen H, Tuck T, Ji X, Zhou X, Kelly G, Cuerrier A, et al. Quality assessment of Japanese knotweed (Fallopia japonica) grown on Prince Edward Island as a source of resveratrol. Journal of Agricultural and Food Chemistry. 2013;**61**(26):6383-6392

[84] Gugleva V, Zasheva S, Hristova M, Andonova V. Topical use of resveratrol:

Technological aspects. Pharmacia. 2020;**67**(2):89-94. DOI: 10.3897/pharmacia.67.e48472

[85] Lim Y, Preshaw P, Lin H, Tan K. Resveratrol and its analogs as functional foods in periodontal disease management. Frontiers in Dental Medicine. 2021;**2**:1-13. DOI: 10.3389/fdmed.2021.636423

Chapter 10

Point-of-Care: A Novel Approach to Periodontal Diagnosis

Nancy Srivastava and Shivendra Rana

Abstract

Being one of the prevalent oral diseases, periodontal disease is marked by the presence of gingival inflammation and periodontal tissue destruction. Recently, there is a paradigm shift in the understanding of periodontal disease; it is now believed to be episodic in nature, showing periods of activity and inactivity. Thereby, posing a challenge for clinicians to diagnose this. Conventional diagnostic methods basically measure past tissue destruction, arising the need for new diagnostic methods that should be able to detect active sites of destruction, predict future progression, and determine the response to the therapy thus, leading to early diagnosis and better cure for the patient. One such advance is the development of point-of-care devices, which are rapid chair-side testing methods. These devices are already in use in healthcare services, a common example being home-used pregnancy test strips. This point-of-care technology is now expanding its arms in periodontics as well, thus simplifying diagnosis and improving the therapeutic outcomes of the patient. In light of the above facts, this chapter throws light on periodontal diagnosis and various commercially available point-of-care devices.

Keywords: biomarkers, genetic testing, antigen-antibody reaction, gingivitis, body fluids

1. Introduction

Oral cavity is the home of numerous microorganisms. Exposed to the outer environment, the oral mucosa is under continuous attack from various pathogens. The immune inflammatory response, which arises due to these pathogens, causes inflammation [1].

Periodontitis, the inflammation of periodontium, is one of the leading oral problems affecting the world. And like any other disease, the earlier it is diagnosed, the better is the prognosis [2].

Traditionally, periodontitis has been diagnosed by probing depth, bleeding on probing, or bone loss by radiographs [3, 4]. All these procedures tell us only the destruction caused by the disease till date and reflect only the clinical phenotype and not the biological phenotype. Knowledge about biologic phenotypes helps in assessing the burden of microbial and inflammatory load, which further affects the progression of periodontitis [1].

With advances in sciences, it has become known that diagnostic processes need to reveal much more than just the disease. It needs to help in locating the sites of active

S. No.	Oral fluid	Test	Kit
1.	Saliva	Biochemical test	Oral fluid nano sensor test
			Electronic taste chip
			Ora quick
			Integrated microfluidic platform for oral Diagnostics
		Microbiological test	My periopath
			OMNIgene
			IAI pado test
2.	Gingival crevicular fluid	Biochemical test	Periogard
			Pocket watch
			Periocheck
			Prognostic
			MMP dipstick test
3.	Plaque	Microbiological test	Perioscan (BANA)
			Evalusite
			Perio 2000
			TOPAS
			Genetic test kits
4.	Living tissue	Genetic test	MyperioID
			Periodontitis susceptibility trait test

Table 1.
Table showing various available point-of-care devices [10].

disease, susceptibility of the patient to disease, future progression of the disease, long-term maintenance, patient response, and microbial challenge [5–7].

Point-of-care (POC) testing can be defined as testing performed close to the patient at the time care is required. POC can revolutionize both periodontal diagnostic and therapy. These tests rely on the detection of a plethora of biomarkers of disease activity. These markers present in saliva, gingival crevicular fluid (GCF), plaque, or living tissue are quantifiable and indicate health and disease [8, 9]. This chapter covers all the latest POC diagnostics available (**Table 1**), which detect markers for periodontal diseases.

2. Point-of-care diagnostics

A good diagnostic marker should always have high specificity and sensitivity [11]. Saliva and GCF are vehicles with great potential to be used in diagnostic tests for various diseases. They are easy to collect and are rich in locally or systemically derived biomarkers of periodontal diseases [10].

2.1 Saliva

Saliva is a bio-fluid that is very useful and easily accessible and can be used to monitor oral and systemic health (**Table 2**) [8]. Most of the biomarkers found in

Markers of periodontal soft tissue inflammation	Markers of alveolar bone loss	Collagen breakdown products
Prostaglandin E2	Alkaline phosphatase	Aspartate aminotransferase
β-glucuronidase	Osteoprotegerin	Alanine aminotransferase
IL-1β	Osteocalcin	TIMPs
IL-6	Collagen telopeptidase	MMPs
Tumor necrosis factor-α	Pyridinoline cross-links of type I collagen	α2-macroglobulin
Matrix metalloproteinase (MMP-8,9&13)	RANKL	
	Osteonectin	

Table 2.
demonstrating the biomarkers present in saliva [10].

blood are also present in saliva (**Table 3**). Moreover, unlike blood, it does not clot or easily spreads infections. However, a disadvantage of saliva is the lower concentration of biomarkers in comparison to serum, thus requires the test to be highly sensitive [12]. Moreover, saliva is also influenced by environmental and psychological factors.

2.1.1 Biochemical tests done on saliva

2.1.1.1 Oral fluid nano sensor test (OFNASET)

It is an ultrasensitive and ultraspecific automated electrochemical detection system for salivary proteins and nucleic acids. This test is an oral cancer screening device that is developed by the University of California, Los Angeles (UCLA) collaborative oral fluid diagnostic research laboratory, led by Dr. David Wong [8, 13]. Four salivary mRNA biomarkers (SAT, ODZ, IL-8, and IL-1b) and two salivary proteomic biomarkers (thioredoxin and IL-8) are detected in the system [14].

2.1.1.2 Electronic test chip

This microchip-based detection system is used for measuring analytes (acids, bases, electrolytes, and proteins) in the solution phase. Antigen-antibody reactions

Test kits	
Oral Fluid Nano Sensor Test	Detection of multiple salivary proteins and nucleic acids.
Electronic Taste Chips	Simultaneously monitor several biomarkers related to periodontal disease
OraQuick	Usually detects HIV 1 and HIV 2
Integrated Microfluidic	Quantification of an oral disease biomarker
Platform for Oral Diagnostics	

Table 3.
Commercially available salivary point-of-care diagnostics [10].

take place on the interior surface of microspheres. The microspheres, increase the surface area and thus, makes it more efficient than ELISA, where the reactions take place on a single layer on the bottom of the well [15].

2.1.1.3 OraQuick

It is the first FDA-approved oral swab in-home test for HIV-1 and HIV-2. It is a stick-like device with a fabric swab and provides results within 20 minutes [14].

2.1.1.4 Integrated microfluidic platform for oral diagnostics (IMPOD)

This kit rapidly measures MMP-8 a biomarker for detection of periodontal disease in saliva and other biomarkers by electrophoretic immunoassay [14].

2.1.2 Microbiological tests done on saliva

2.1.2.1 My periopath

My periopath is a commercially available POC device produced by oral DNA labs. It detects the pathogens causing periodontal disease in saliva samples. This test uses DNA polymerase chain reaction to detect the type and concentration of bacteria present in the salivary samples [16].

2.1.2.2 OMNIgene

This kit provides results in a short period and also these results can be mailed or faxed to the clinician. It can identify pathogens by either DNA probe or RNA probe. By DNA probes, it identifies *Porphyromonas gingivalis, Prevotella intermedia, Aggregatibacter actinomycetemcomitans, Fusobacterium nucleatum, Eikenella corrodens, Campylobacter rectus, Bacteroides forsythus,* and *Treponema denticola* [17]. By RNA probe, it identifies *Aggregatibacter actinomycetemcomitans, Porphyromonas gingivalis, Treponema forsythia,* and *Treponema denticola* [16]. OMNIgene-ORAL is a commercial POC device produced by DNA Genotek company.

2.2 Gingival crevicular fluid (GCF)

GCF is a body fluid derived from serum, leukocytes, and cells of periodontium and oral microflora [18]. Its composition is influenced by both external environment and body physiology [19]. Therefore, GCF contains a variety of potential markers derived from the host and bacteria from supragingival and subgingival plaque (**Table 4**). These biomarkers can be categorized as (i) inflammatory and immune products, (ii) bacterial enzymes, (iii) host-derived enzymes, (iv) tissue breakdown products, and (v) bone-specific proteins.

The biomarkers in GCF provide information regarding inflammation, loss of bone, patient susceptibility, detection of periodontal disease, prognosis of disease, and onset of disease (**Table 5**) [20, 21]. The disadvantages of GCF are that it requires multiple samples of individual tooth sites and extreme lab processing [22]. Moreover, the collection of samples is difficult, and easy contamination of GCF can occur [23]. This makes GCF a difficult medium for chair-side diagnosis.

Inflammatory and immune products	Bacterial proteases	Host-derived enzymes	Tissue breakdown products	Bone-specific proteins
Prostaglandin E2 (PGE2)	Alkaline phosphatase	Alkaline phosphatase	Glycosaminoglycan	Pyridinium crosslink urine pyridinoline
Cytokines	Aminopeptidases	β-Glucuronidase	Hyaluronic acid	Pyridinium crosslink collagen peptide fragment
Antibacterial antibodies	Chondroitin sulfatase	Elastase	Chondroitin-4-sulfate	Tartrate-resistant acid phosphatase
Acute-phase proteins	Collagenase	Cathepsins	Chondroitin-6-sulfate	Hydroxyproline
Complement	Fibrinolysin	Serine proteinase (G)	Dermatan sulfate	Galactosyl hydroxylysine
Vasoactive intestinal peptide	Glucosidases	Nonspecific neutral proteinases	Hydroxyproline	Glycosaminoglycans
Neurokinin a	Hemolysin	Matrix metalloproteinase-1,3,8,13	Fibronectin fragments	Osteonectin and bone phosphoprotein
Neopterin	Hyaluronidase	Aspartate amino transferase	Connective tissue and bone proteins	osteocalcin
Platelet-activating factor	Phospholipase	Myeloperoxidases	Type I collagen peptides	
	Hydroxyproline	Lactate dehydrogenase	polypeptide growth factor	

Table 4.
Biomarkers in gingival crevicular fluid [10].

Test kits	Enzymes
Periogard	AST
Pocket watch	AST
Periocheck	Collagenase (neutral protease)
Prognostik (Dentsply), Biolise	Elastase (serine protease)
MMP dipstick method	MMP

Table 5.
Commercially available kits using GCF for detecting host-derived enzymes [10].

2.2.1 Biochemical tests done on GCF

2.2.1.1 Periogard

It detects aspartate aminotransferase (AST), which is released on cell death due to periodontal diseases (**Figure 1**) [24]. Thus, periogard can easily locate sites with active disease processes [25]. The only disadvantage is the numerous steps required and difficulty in colour measurement [26].

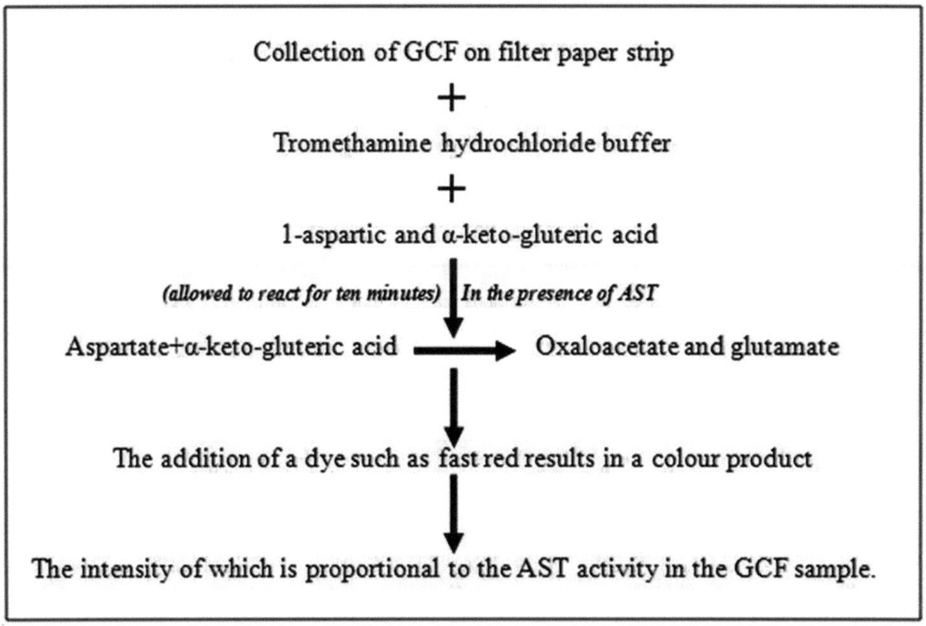

Figure 1.
Principle of periogard.

2.2.1.2 Pocket watch

Pocket watch also analyzes AST levels but through a different method. AST acts as a catalyst in the exchange of an amino group of cysteine sulfuric acid by α-keto-gluteric acid to produce β-sulfinyl pyruvate in the presence of pyridoxal phosphate. Inorganic sulfite is released by the spontaneous decomposition of glutamate β-sulfinyl pyruvate. These sulfite ions produced react with malachite green to convert it into a colorless form, thereby showing the pink-colored rhodamine B dye. Thus, the rate of conversion assesses the AST concentration [27].

2.2.1.3 Periocheck

It detects neutral proteases in GCF, such as elastases, proteinases, and collagenases, and is a FDA-approved rapid chair-side test (**Figure 2**) [28].

2.2.1.4 Prognostik

It was developed in 1993 and helped in identifying active sites by measuring elevated MMP (**Figure 3**). MMPs are host-derived proteinases, which play a major role in periodontitis and dental peri-implant health and disease. MMPs, such as elastases, are released by the lysosomes of polymorphonuclear leukocytes [29].

2.2.1.5 MMP dipstick

MMP dipstick detects MMP-8, which differentiates sites having healthy gingiva, gingivitis, and periodontitis [30].

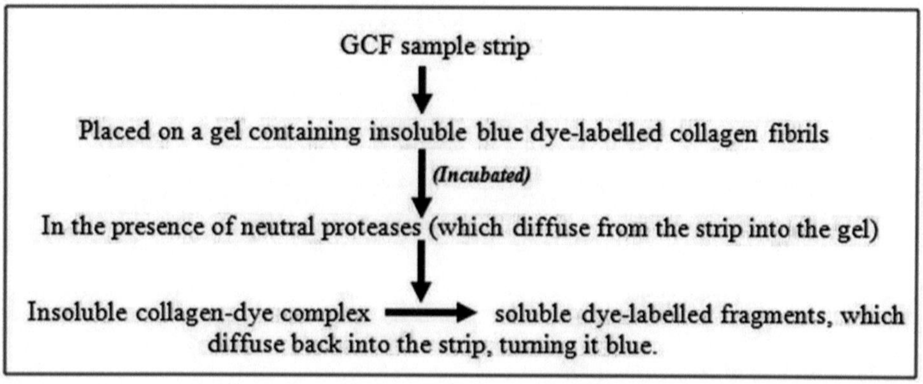

Figure 2.
Principle of periocheck.

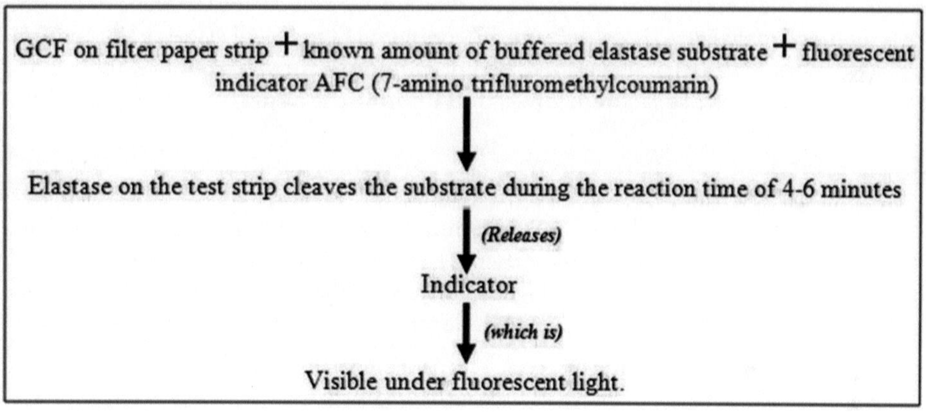

Figure 3.
Principle of prognostik.

Markers present in dental biofilm		
Specific	**Nonspecific**	**Systemic**
Immunoglobulins (IgA, IgG and IgM)	Mucins	C-reactive protein
	Lysozyme	
	Lactoferrin	
	Histatin	
	Peroxidase	

Table 6.
Biomarkers present in dental biofilm [10].

2.2.1.6 Plaque

Numerous studies have detected pathogens in dental plaque causing periodontal diseases (**Table 6**). Numerous commercially available kits have emerged, which detect these pathogens and help in diagnosis and treatment (**Table 7**) [10].

Test kits	Bacteria and their products
Perioscan (BANA test)	Trypsin like protease
Oral B lab	
Evalusite (Kodak)	*P.gingivalis, P.intermedia, A.actinomycetemcomitans*
Perioscan/ Diamond probe/Probe 2000 system	For volatile sulfur compounds
TOPAS	Bacterial toxins and protease

Table 7.
Other commercially available kits for detecting bacterial protease [10].

2.2.2 Microbial tests done on plaque

2.2.2.1 Perioscan (BANA)

It basically detects trypsin-like proteins, which are produced by various periopathogens, such as *P. gingivalis*, *T. denticola,* and *T. forsythia* (**Figure 4**) [31]. A major disadvantage of perioscan is that it cannot differentiate among these bacteria. Moreover, it cannot detect non-trypsin-like enzymes, thus limiting the number of pathogens [32].

2.2.2.2 Evalusite

This kit uses membrane-based enzyme immunoassay and can detect *A. actinomycetemcomitans, P. gingivalis, and P. intermedia* (**Figure 5**). The major limitation is the ability to detect only these three pathogens. Moreover, the detection is done by assessing the change in color, which is always subjective and varies from person to person [24].

2.2.2.3 Perio 2000

Similar to perioscan, this kit detects *P. gingivali, P. intermedia,* and *T. forsythia.* It measures volatile sulfide compounds (VSCs), which are produced by bacteria after

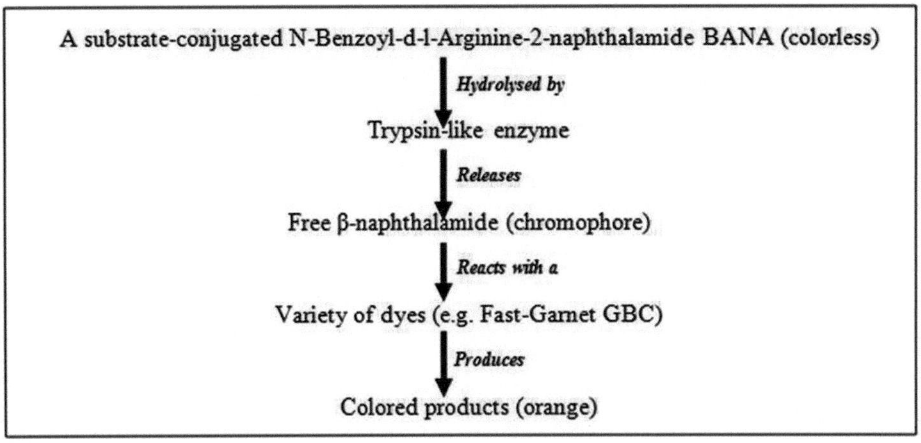

Figure 4.
Principle of perioscan.

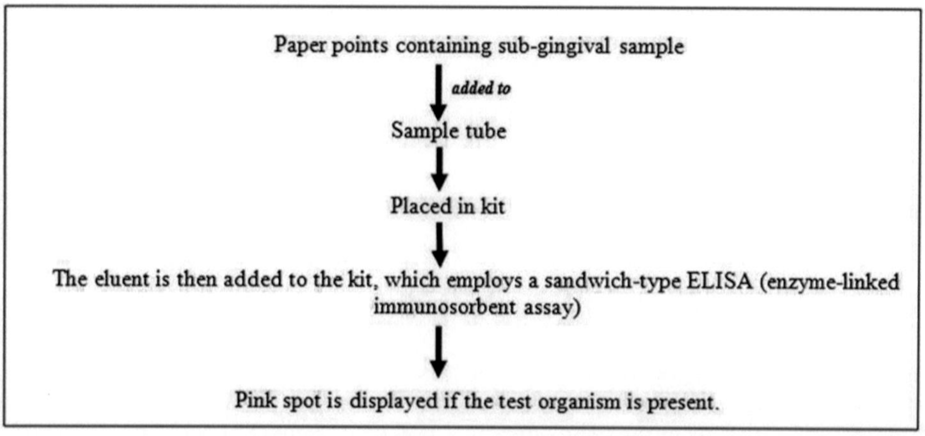

Figure 5.
Principle of evalusite.

degrading the serum proteins (cysteine and methionine), and displays it digitally. The main advantage is that there is no need to collect GCF as the probe tip can be inserted directly into the gingival sulcus.

2.2.2.1 Toxicity prescreening assay (TOPAS)

It directly detects bacterial toxins and bacterial proteins in GCF. Thus, it is able to locate active disease sites. It is a chair-side test kit that shows results by changing color intensity according to toxin concentration in the GCF [33].

2.2.3 Genetic tests

2.2.3.1 MyperioID

MyperioID does not identify any pathogens, but basically provides genetic susceptibility of the patient to periodontal diseases [16].

2.2.3.2 Periodontitis susceptibility trait test

The periodontitis susceptibility trait test (PST) is the test that identifies the genetic predisposition of the patient for periodontitis. It detects polymorphism in IL-1 gene, which has been linked with periodontal diseases [17].

2.3 Diagnostics-lab-on-chip

Lab-on-chip is a newer generation of POC technology still undergoing development [14]. It basically integrates and automates all the complexities of a laboratory procedure onto a computer chip [28]. This technology will thus measure multiple biomarkers in a small sample of plaque, GCF, or saliva [13, 16]. It will omit all the requirements of heavy expensive equipment or trained lab technicians. The result will be chair-side, instant, and not subjective.

3. Advantages of POC

It increases patient cooperation as no blood is drawn from the patient. Cost and inventory for shipping samples to a centralized laboratory are reduced. Large populations can be screened. Treatment can be started immediately as results are obtained rapidly. It requires lesser training and resources than current diagnostic methods. Patients with higher risk can be recognized and treated.

4. Disadvantages of POC

The use of POC diagnostics in periodontal surveillance looks promising; however, in the clinical setting, these approaches suffer from various obstacles. These tests still need validation and acceptance by dentists. Cost-effectiveness of the procedure and kit is another concern. Finally, the clinician needs to be abreast with the knowledge of diagnosis, disease risks, and prevention before diagnostics may be integrated into routine clinical periodontal practice.

5. Conclusion

The cornerstone for a successful periodontal treatment is an accurate initial diagnosis. The current existing diagnostic methods suffice the purpose but cannot achieve any more goals than this. Knowledge of patient susceptibility and active disease sites are desired by any clinician from the diagnostic methods. With the introduction of new chair-side test kits, which use the host and bacterial markers of periodontal disease, monitoring of specific sites is now possible. The various oral fluids easily available for test are under great amount of research and investigation. Though with various challenges, saliva, GCF, and plaque are promising mediums to be used for periodontal diseases. One of the latest clinical applications of POCT is in the detection of the SARS-CoV-2 virus. Although SARS-CoV-2 RNA detection in nasopharyngeal swabs is reported to be the gold standard method but it is an invasive method, and therefore uncomfortable for the patient. Due to the limitations of this method, saliva is now suggested to be a better alternative because it is easy to collect the sample and is not uncomfortable for the patient [34]. SpeciMAX is the commercially available saliva collection kit for the detection of SARS-CoV-2 virus.

The need of an hour is to develop POC devices for diseases, such as cancer and hyperthyroidism, so that these can be detected with the help of biomarkers at home leading to their early diagnosis and effective intervention at right time.

Author details

Nancy Srivastava[1*] and Shivendra Rana[2]

1 Department of Periodontics, NIMS Dental College and Hospital, Jaipur, Rajasthan, India

2 Department of Oral and Maxillofacial Pathology, Rajasthan Dental College, Jaipur, Rajasthan, India

*Address all correspondence to: dr.nancy15@gmail.com

References

[1] Hernández M, Vernal R, Sorsa T, Tervahartiala T, Mäntylä P, Gamonal J. The role of immuno-inflammatory response in the pathogenesis of chronic periodontitis and development of chair-side point of care diagnostics. In: Buduneli N, editor. Pathogenesis and Treatment of Periodontitis [Internet]. London: InTech Publishing Co; 2012 [cited 2022 Oct 09]. Available from: https://www.intechopen.com/chapters/26476 doi: 10.5772/32658

[2] Lee Y, Wong DT. Saliva: An emerging biofluid for early detection of disease. American Journal of Dentistry. 2009;**22**:241-248

[3] Sahingur SE, Cohen RE. Analysis of host responses and risk for disease progression. Periodontology. 2000;**34**:57-83

[4] Position paper: Diagnosis of periodontal disease. Journal of Periodontology. 2003;**74**:1237-1247

[5] Offenbacher S. Periodontal diseases: Pathogenesis. Annals of Periodontology. 1996;**1**:821-878

[6] Giannobile WV, Beikler T, Kinney JS, Ramseier CA, Morelli T, Wong DT. Saliva as a diagnostic tool for periodontal disease: Current state and future directions. Periodontology. 2000;**2009**(50):52-64

[7] Chapple I. Periodontal disease diagnosis: Current status and future developments. Journal of Dentistry. 1997;**25**:3-15

[8] Spielmann N, Wong DT. Saliva: Diagnostics and therapeutic perspectives. Oral Diseases. 2011;**17**:345-354

[9] Wei F, Wong DT. Point-of-care platforms for salivary diagnostics. The Chinese Journal of Dental Research. 2012;**15**:7-15

[10] Taba M Jr, Kinney J, Kim AS, Giannobile WV. Diagnostic biomarkers for oral and periodontal diseases. Dental Clinics of North America. 2005;**49**:551-572

[11] Loos BG, Tjoa S. Host-derived diagnostic markers for periodontitis: Do they exist in gingival crevice fluid? Periodontology. 2000;**39**:53-72

[12] Miller SM. Saliva testing: A non-traditional diagnostic tool. Clinical Laboratory Science. 1994;**7**:3944

[13] Wong DT. Salivaomics. Journal of American Dental Association. 2012;**143**:19S-24S

[14] Priyanka N, Kalra N, Shanbhag N, Kumar K, Seema BB, et al. Recent approaches in saliva as a credible periodontal diagnostic and prognostic marker. AOSR. 2012;**2**:40-46

[15] Christodoulides N, Tran M, Floriano PN, et al. A microchip-based multianalyte assay system for the assessment of cardiac risk. Analytical Chemistry. 2002;**74**:3030-3036

[16] Chepuri T, Gooty JR, Durvasala S, Palaparthi R. Chair side diagnostic test kits in periodontics. Indian Journal of Dental Advances. 2015;**7**:41-45

[17] Pajnigara NG, Kolte AP, Kolte RA, Pajnigara NG. Chair side diagnostic kits in Periodontics. International Dental Journal Of Student's Research. 2016;**4**:25-31

[18] Uitto V-J. Gingival crevice fluid – an introduction. Periodontology. 2000;**2003**(31):9-11

[19] Champagne CME, Buchanan W. Potential for gingival crevice fluid measures as predictors of risk for periodontal diseases. Periodontology. 2000;**2003**(31):167-180

[20] Zia A, Khan S, Bey A, Gupta ND, Mukhtar-Un-Nisar S. Oral biomarkers in the diagnosis and progression of periodontal diseases. Biology and Medicine. 2011;**3**:45-52

[21] Chapple I. Periodontal diagnosis and treatment -- where does the future lie? Periodontology. 2000;**51**:9-24

[22] Patil PB, Patil BR. Saliva: A diagnostic biomarker of periodontal diseases. Journal of Indian Society Periodontology. 2011;**15**:310-317

[23] Persson G, De Rouen T, Page R. Relationship between levels of aspartate aminotransferase in gingival crevicular fluid and active tissue destruction in treated chronic periodontitis patients. Journal of Periodontal Research. 1990;**25**:81-87

[24] Mikx FH, Renggli HH. How sensible are bacteriological tests in periodontology? Nederlands Tijdschrift voor Tandheelkunde. 1994;**101**:484-488

[25] Chambers D, Imrey P, Cohen R, Crawford J, Alves M, Mcswiggin T. A longitudinal study of aspartate aminotransferase in human gingival crevicular fluid. Journal of Periodontal Research. 1991;**26**:65-74

[26] Persson GR, Alves M, Chambers D, et al. A multicentered clinical trial of PerioGard in distinguishing between diseased and healthy periodontal sites. Journal of Clinical Periodontology. 1995;**22**:794-803

[27] Shimhadaka K, Mizuno T. Analysis of AST in gingival crevicular fluid assessed using Perio Watch: A longitudinal study with initial therapy. Journal of Clinical Periodontology. 2000;**27**:819-823

[28] Chapple I, Matthews J, Thorpe G, Glenwright H, Smith J, Saxby M. A new ultrasensitive chemiluminescent assay for the site-specific quantification of alkaline phosphatase in gingival crevicular fluid. Journal of Periodontal Research. 1993;**28**:266-273

[29] Armitage G, Jeffcoat M, Chadwick D, et al. Longitudinal evaluation of elastase as a marker for the progression of periodontitis. Journal of Periodontology. 1994;**65**:120

[30] Sorsa T et al. Collagenase-2 (MMP-8) as a point-of-care biomarker in periodontitis and cardiovascular diseases. Therapeutic response to non-antimicrobial properties of tetracyclines. Pharmacological Research. 2011;**63**:108-113

[31] Laughton B, Syned S, Loesche W. API ZYM system for identification of Bacteroides ssp., Capnocytophagia ssp., and spirochaetes of oral origin. Journal of Clinical Microbiology. 1982;**15**:97-127

[32] Loesche W, Syed S, Stoll J. Trypsin-like activity in sub-gingival plaque: A diagnostic marker for spirochetes and periodontal disease? Journal of Periodontology. 1987;**58**:266-273

[33] Puscasu CG, Dumitriu A, Dumitriu HT. Biochemical and enzymatic diagnosis aids in periodontal disease. OHDMBSC. 2005;**4**:19-25

[34] Caixeta DC, Oliveira SW, et al. One-year update on salivary diagnostic of COVID-19. Frontiers in Public Health. 2021;**9**:589-564